GROW

Paul DeMayo readies himself for a set of
high-intensity lateral raises.

35

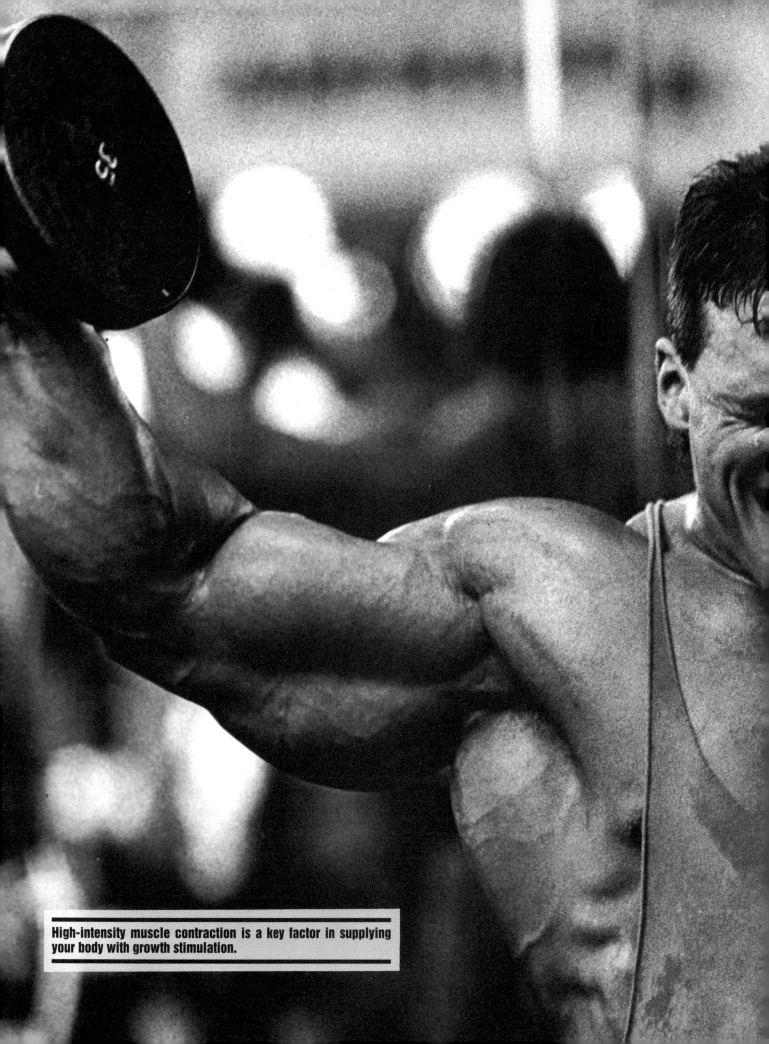

High-intensity muscle contraction is a key factor in supplying your body with growth stimulation.

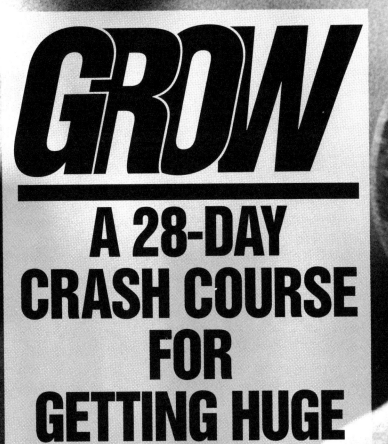

GROW

A 28-DAY CRASH COURSE FOR GETTING HUGE

ELLINGTON DARDEN, PH.D.
PHOTOS BY CHRIS LUND

CB

CONTEMPORARY
BOOKS

CHICAGO

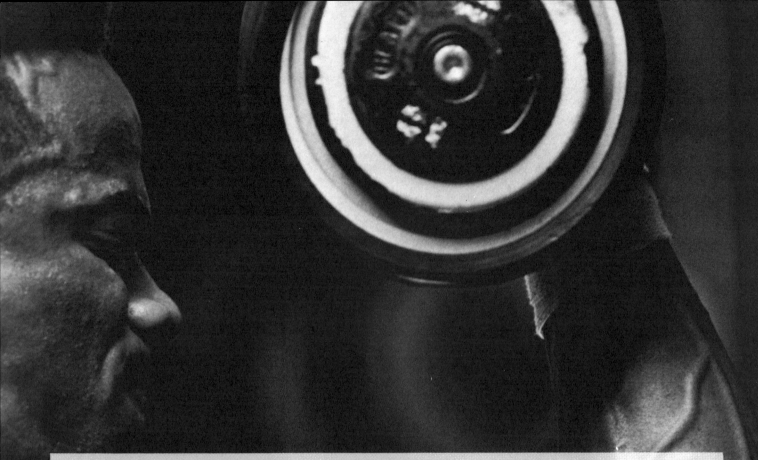

Library of Congress Cataloging-in-Publication Data

Darden, Ellington
Grow: a 28-day crash course for getting huge / Ellington Darden :
photos by Chris Lund.
p.   cm.
ISBN 0-8092-3802-0
1. Bodybuilding.   I. Title
GV546.5.D3545   1993
646.7'5—dc20

Cover design by Martin Moskof
Book design: Martin Moskof
Book design assistant: George Brady

WARNING!
The high-intensity routines in this book are intended only for
healthy men and women. People with health problems should not
follow these routines without a physician's approval. Before
beginning any exercise or dietary program, always consult with
your doctor.

Other Books of Interest by Ellington Darden, Ph.D.

BIG
Massive Muscles in 10 Weeks
Super High-Intensity Bodybuilding
The Nautilus Diet
How to Lose Body Fat
Conditioning for Football
The Nautilus Book
The Nautilus Nutrition Book
The Nautilus Woman
The Nautilus Bodybuilding Book
The Nautilus Advanced Bodybuilding Book
The Six-Week Fat-to-Muscle Makeover
Big Arms in Six Weeks
100 High-Intensity Ways to Improve Your Bodybuilding
32 Days to a 32-Inch Waist
Hot Hips and Fabulous Thighs
Two Weeks to a Tighter Tummy
New High-Intensity Bodybuilding
Bigger Muscles in 42 Days
High-Intensity Strength Training

For a free catalog of Dr. Darden's books, please send a self-
addressed, stamped envelope to Nautilus Sports/Medical
Industries, P.O. Box 160, Independence, VA 24348.

Front cover photo of Jim Quinn and back cover photo of Paul
Dillett by Chris Lund. All interior photos by Chris Lund, except as
noted: Ken Hutchins: 86 bottom, 87 bottom, 91, 106, 107 right,
133, 141, 148/ Walter Coker: 122, 123, 126, 127, 130, 131, 134,
135, 138, 139, 142, 143, 146, 147, 150, 151, 154, 155/ Ellington
Darden: 184, 185, 187

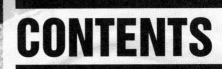

CONTENTS

Mike Matarazzo knows that strict, slow repetitions involve more muscle fibers.

Right: Alq Gurley contracts his shapely arm.

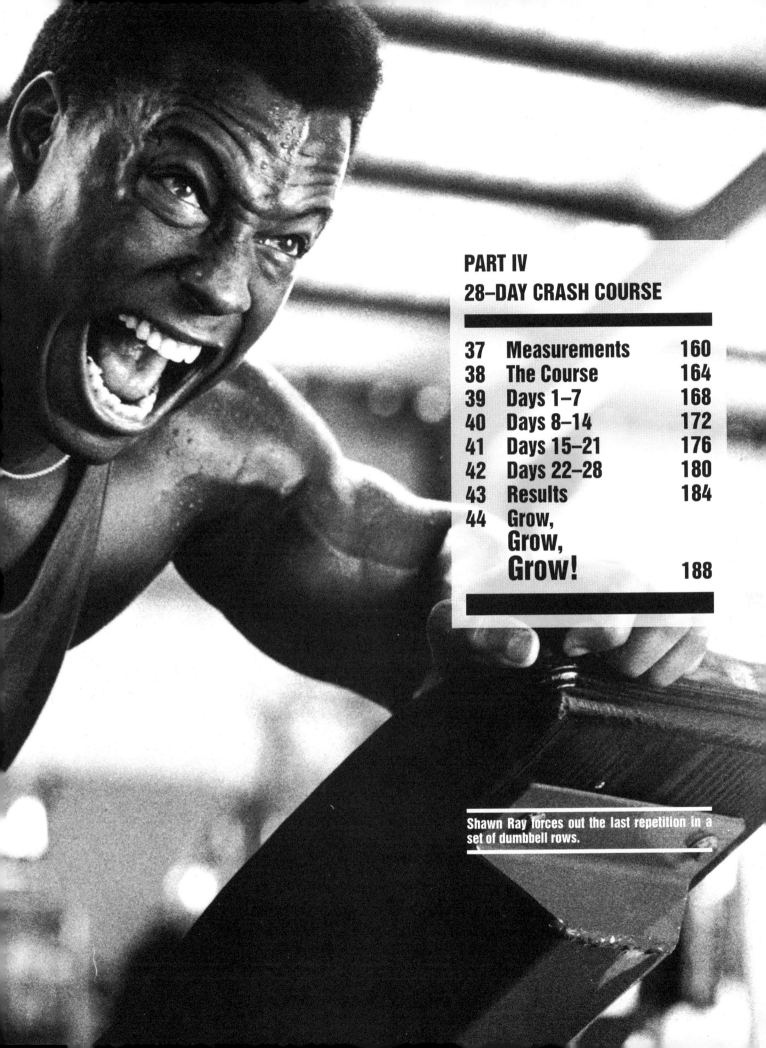

PART IV
28–DAY CRASH COURSE

Shawn Ray forces out the last repetition in a set of dumbbell rows.

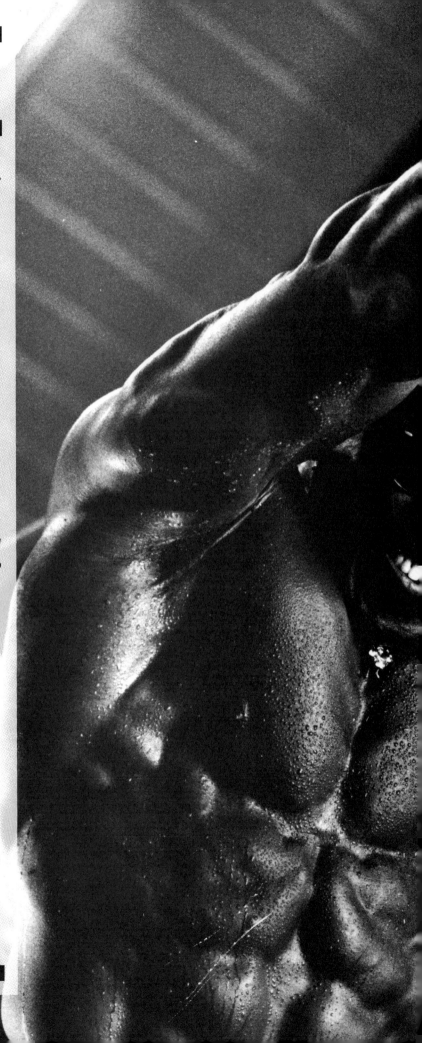

GROW NOW!

So you want to grow. You want to add mass to your frame. You want bigger and stronger muscles.

Millions of teenagers each year join the ranks of young men who desire to get bigger. Most, though, fail in their quest for larger and stronger muscles. They fail because they become mesmerized by what they see and read in the glossy muscle magazines.

Most of the training articles, which allegedly are authored by a current champion, are actually ghostwritten in-house by staff writers and editors. These people are experts with words, phrases, and rhetoric to get your attention and ultimately get you to buy the magazine's mail-order products.

These articles are filled with exaggerated claims and supposedly never-before-revealed training secrets. Unfortunately, if the advice is taken at face value and followed, the end result could be downright dangerous.

The vast majority of young bodybuilders do <u>not</u> have the muscle structure nor the recovery ability to perform the recommended marathon, triple-split training sessions. The result is often that many bodybuilders become smaller and weaker rather than bigger and stronger.

What does it take to get your muscles to grow? In very simple terms, it takes

- Hard
- Brief
- Progressive
- Slow
- Infrequent

exercise combined with proper eating and adequate resting.

This simple approach is illustrated and described in the next 44 chapters. In fact, the last eight chapters present the exact 28-day crash course that Jeff Turner—a 19-year-old athlete—used to add more than 20 pounds of mass to his muscular body.

If you're willing to follow directions precisely, and if you're willing to work harder but briefer, then this manual is for you.

Get ready for your body to GROW!

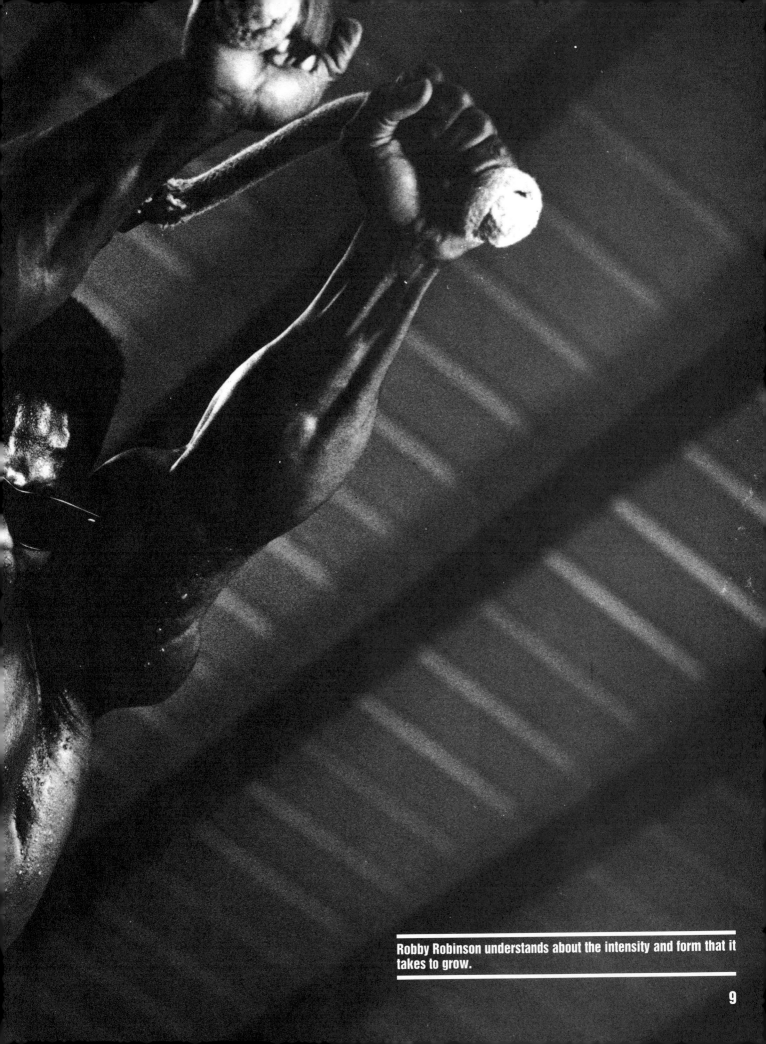

Robby Robinson understands about the intensity and form that it takes to grow.

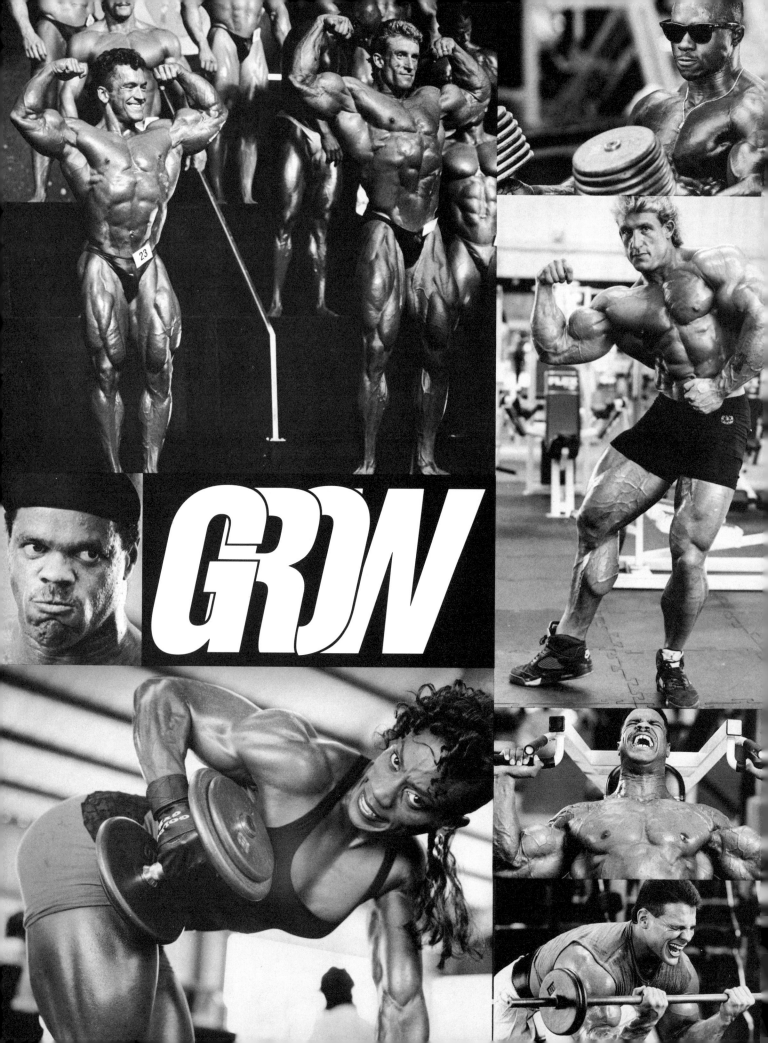

GROW

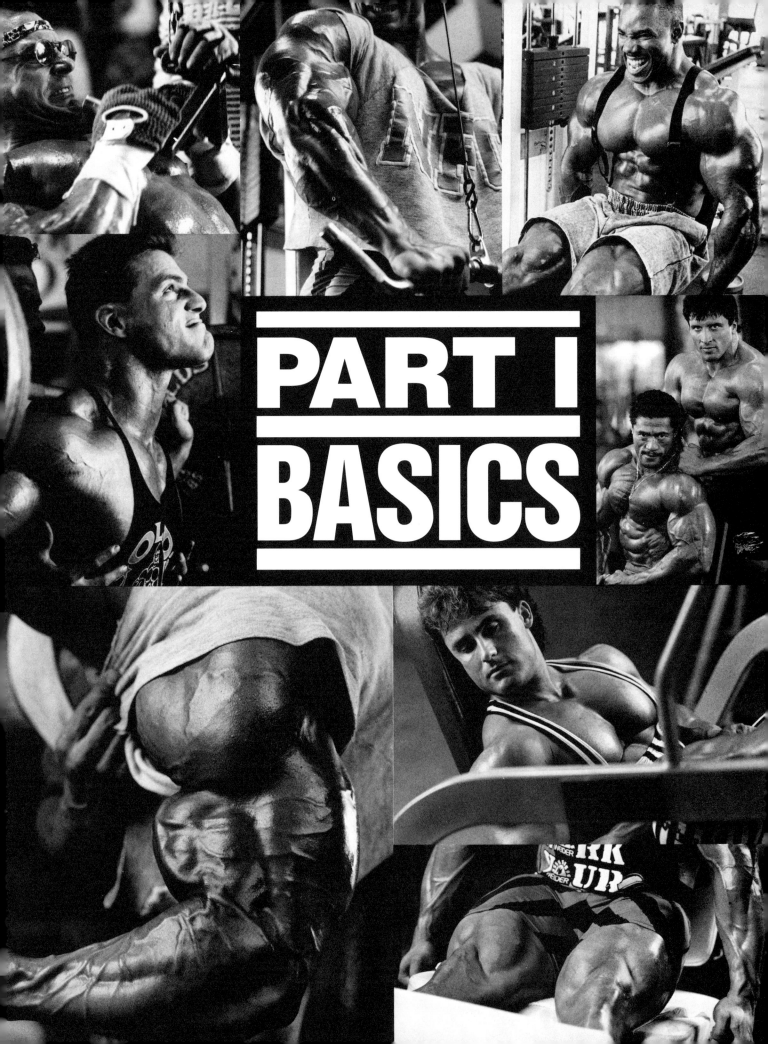

PART I
BASICS

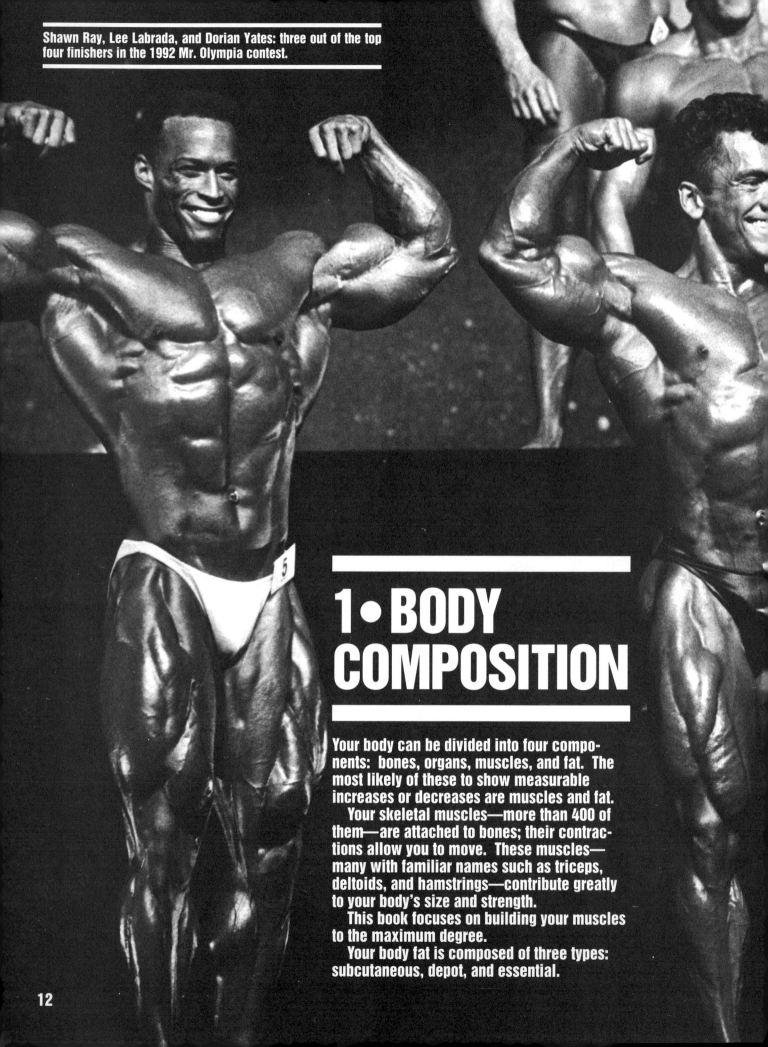

Shawn Ray, Lee Labrada, and Dorian Yates: three out of the top four finishers in the 1992 Mr. Olympia contest.

1• BODY COMPOSITION

Your body can be divided into four components: bones, organs, muscles, and fat. The most likely of these to show measurable increases or decreases are muscles and fat.

Your skeletal muscles—more than 400 of them—are attached to bones; their contractions allow you to move. These muscles—many with familiar names such as triceps, deltoids, and hamstrings—contribute greatly to your body's size and strength.

This book focuses on building your muscles to the maximum degree.

Your body fat is composed of three types: subcutaneous, depot, and essential.

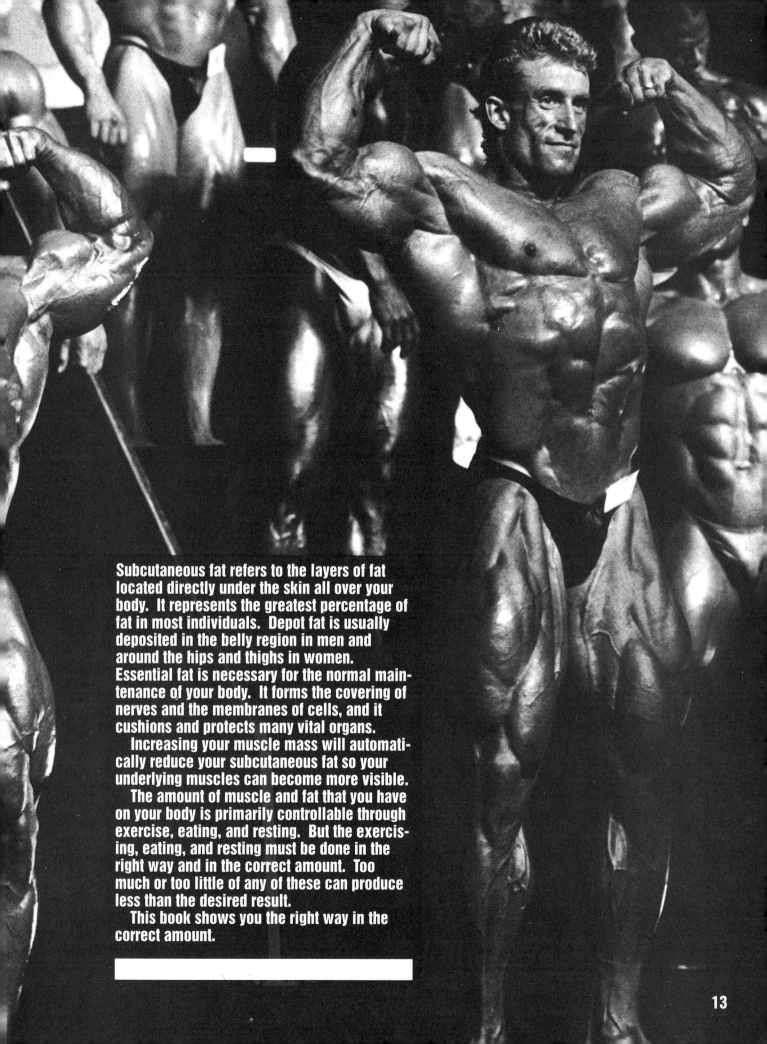

Subcutaneous fat refers to the layers of fat located directly under the skin all over your body. It represents the greatest percentage of fat in most individuals. Depot fat is usually deposited in the belly region in men and around the hips and thighs in women. Essential fat is necessary for the normal maintenance of your body. It forms the covering of nerves and the membranes of cells, and it cushions and protects many vital organs.

Increasing your muscle mass will automatically reduce your subcutaneous fat so your underlying muscles can become more visible.

The amount of muscle and fat that you have on your body is primarily controllable through exercise, eating, and resting. But the exercising, eating, and resting must be done in the right way and in the correct amount. Too much or too little of any of these can produce less than the desired result.

This book shows you the right way in the correct amount.

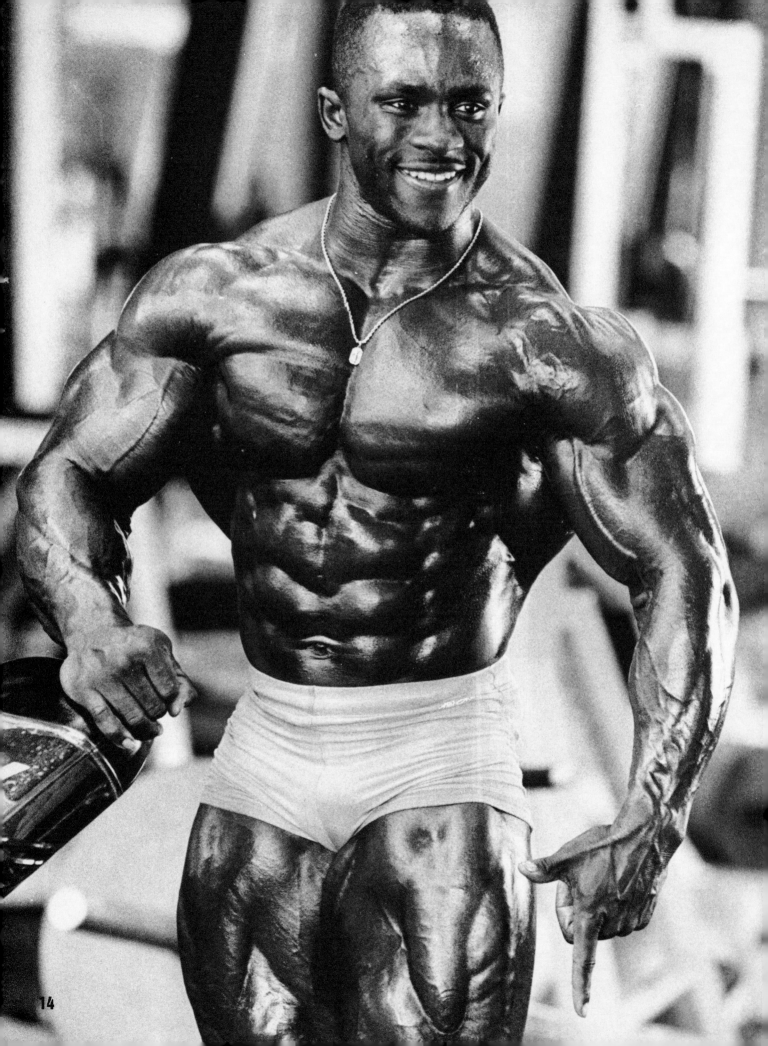

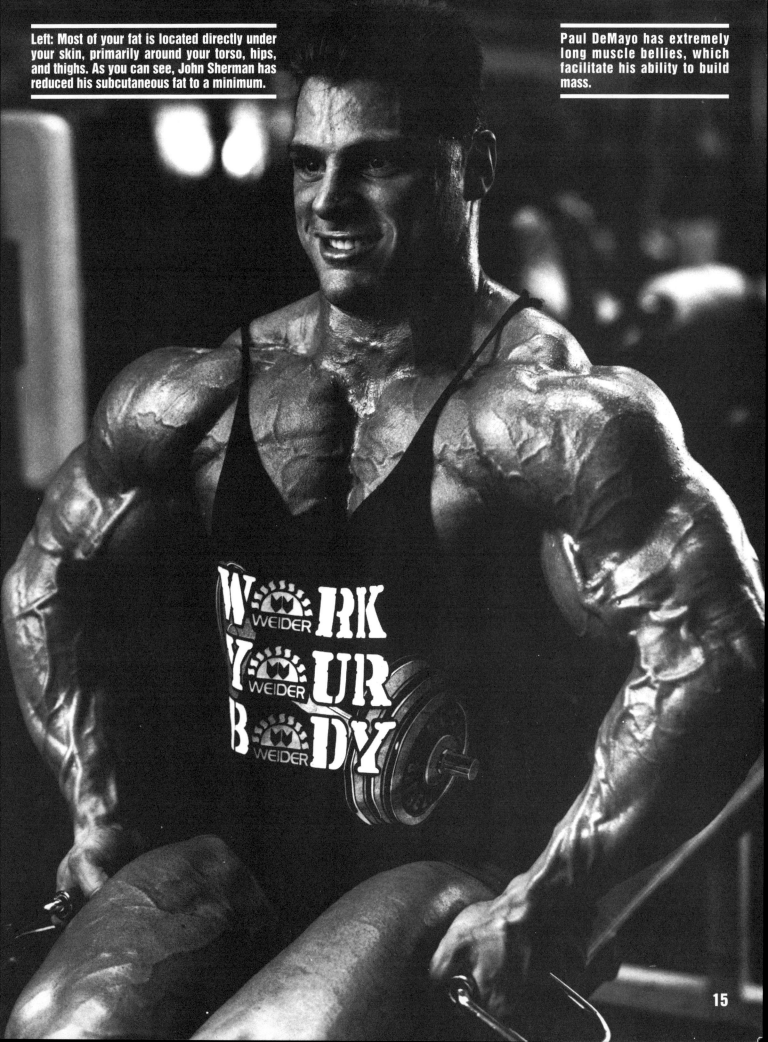

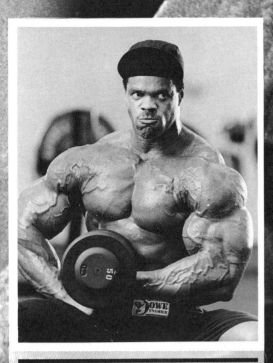

Paul Dillett has some of the most massive, well-defined muscles in bodybuilding today.

2 • MUSCLE

Here are some interesting facts about muscles that will help you apply the guidelines offered in this manual.

■ Exercise, if properly performed, provides a stimulus for muscle growth. If given adequate rest and proper nutrition, the stimulated muscle responds by developing more actin and myosin protein filaments. The increase in these filaments produces larger and stronger muscles.

■ Small projections called cross-bridges extend from the myosin filaments to the surrounding actin filaments during muscle contraction. Repeating contractile units are called sarcomeres. Many sarcomeres form a myofibril, which is the thread running throughout the muscles. Groups of myofibrils are bound together by membranes called sarcolemmas to form individual muscle fibers. Muscle fibers are surrounded by sheaths called perimysia into bundles of fibers known as fasciculi. These bundles of fibers are bound by connective tissue called

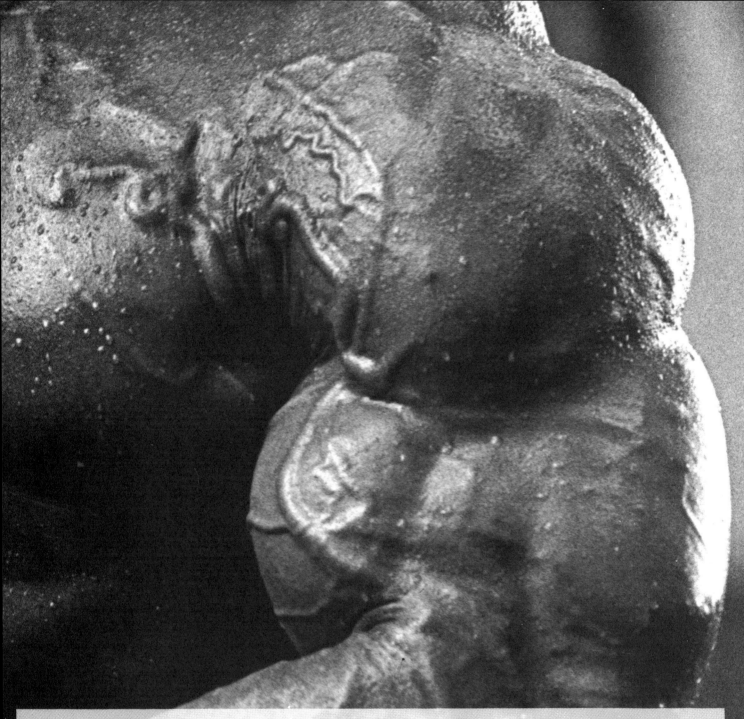

epimysia and function together as a specific muscle, such as the pectoralis major.

■ When a muscle is activated, it produces tension and attempts to shorten; in other words, it tends to pull its attachments closer together. It should be understood, however, that muscle contraction actually means muscle tension and does not necessarily mean a change in length. A working muscle may shorten, lengthen, or remain the same.

■ Prime-mover muscles are responsible for performing a given movement. For example, the biceps of your upper arms are the prime movers for elbow flexion.

Antagonist muscles are responsible for performing the opposite movement of the prime movers. For example, your triceps are the prime-mover muscles for elbow extension, which makes them antagonists to your biceps.

To perform an elbow flexion exercise your biceps (prime movers) must contract and shorten, while your triceps (antagonists) must relax and lengthen. Fortunately, these muscles function simultaneously: biceps contraction is stimulated and triceps involvement is inhibited.

■ A concentric, or positive, contraction results when a muscle exerts force and shortens. Thus, the muscle force is greater than the resistance force. Since the muscle-shortening process involves fric-

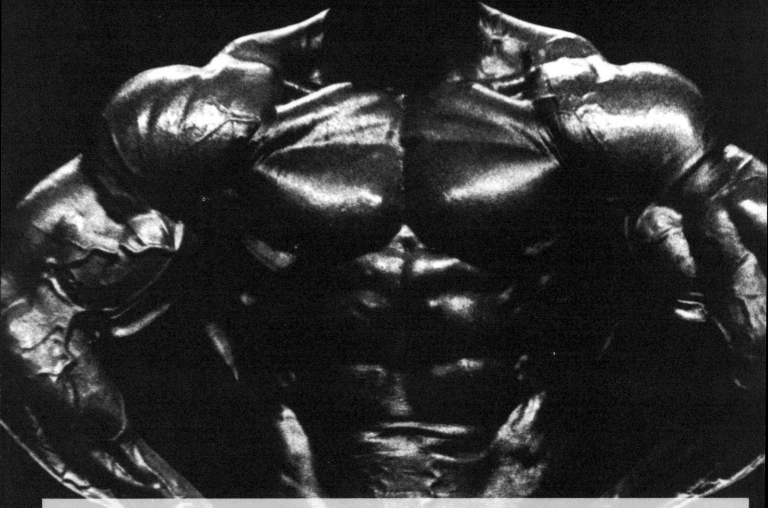

tion, the effective muscle-force output is decreased by approximately 20 percent. For example, you are able to hold a 100-pound barbell at 90 degrees of elbow flexion, but you are able to lift positively an 80-pound barbell. Due to friction working against you, the 100 pounds of muscle-force input is decreased to 80 pounds of muscle-force output.

■ An eccentric, or negative, contraction results when a muscle exerts force and lengthens, as in a lowering movement. Thus, the muscle force is less than the resistance force. Once again, friction is involved, but this time the effective muscle force is <u>increased</u> by approximately 20 percent. For example, you are able to hold a 100-pound barbell at 90

degrees of elbow flexion, but you can lower negatively a 120-pound barbell. Due to friction working for you, the 100 pounds of muscle-force input is elevated to 120 pounds of muscle-force output.

Review these facts about muscle stimulation, prime movers, and positive and negative contraction. They are important in the growth process.

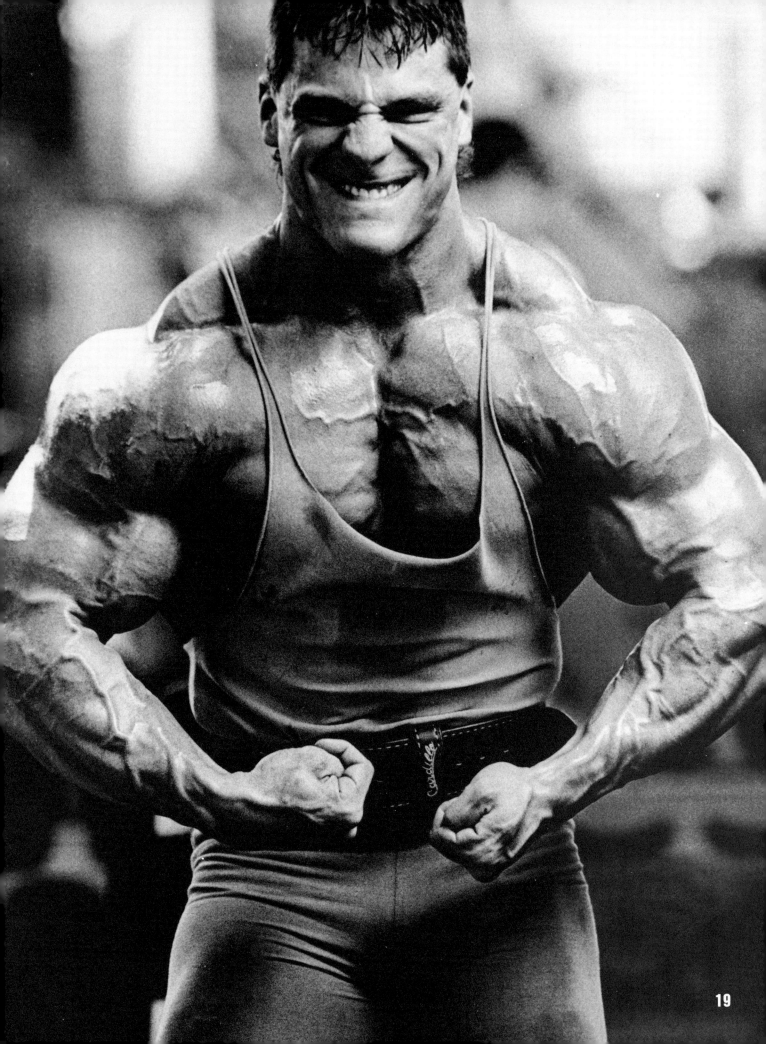

3 • STIMULATION

More than 20 years ago Dr. Alfred Goldberg and his colleagues at Harvard University made a significant discovery about muscle growth. They found that if a muscle is stimulated to grow, it will grow— period. It will grow in spite of a lack of food, rest, growth hormone, and insulin.

Stimulation is the primary factor in the growth process. And stimulation is a result of exercise, pure and simple—the right type of exercise.

Yes, it is true that many other factors facilitate optimum growth. But without the initial stimulation at the cellular level, nothing happens.

The remaining chapters in Part I describe the parameters of ideal exercise.

It takes heavy resistance to stimulate your muscles to grow.

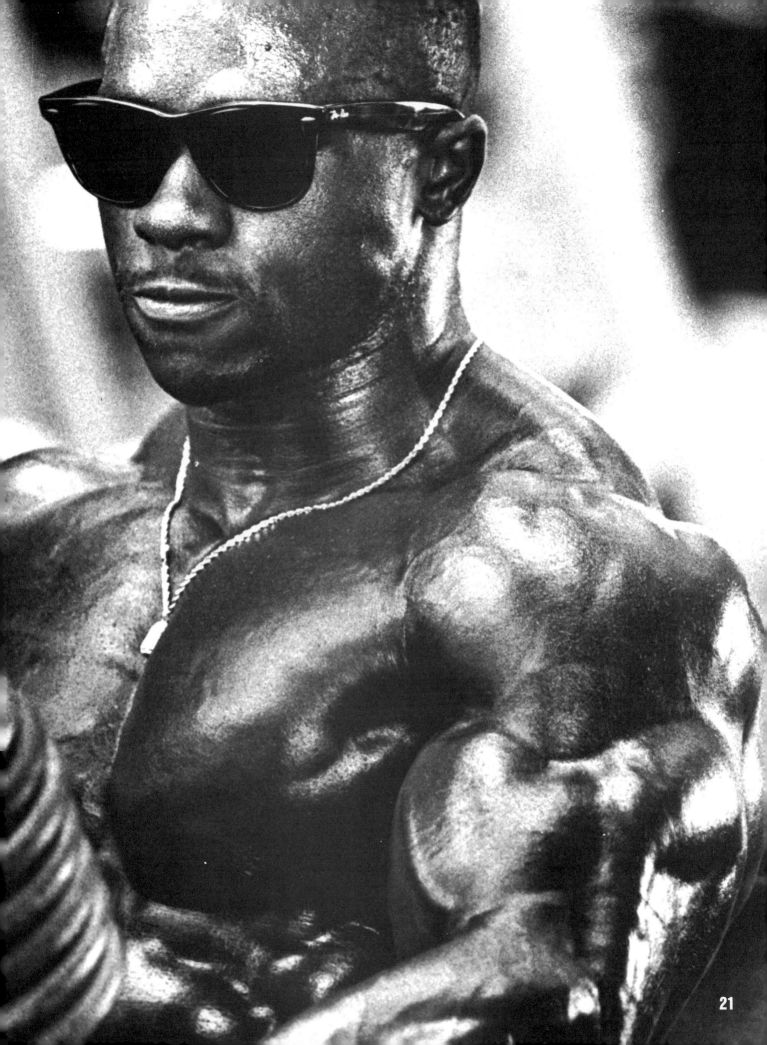

4 • INTENSITY

The intensity of your exercise must be high for optimum muscle stimulation. High-intensity exercise means continuing a movement until your muscles can no longer contract positively. This state is often referred to as momentary muscle fatigue, because your involved muscles have reached their temporary functional limit. Reaching momentary muscular fatigue on each exercise is an important aspect of the muscle-growth process.

Yet many bodybuilders seem to go to great lengths to avoid intense exercise. The intensity of each exercise is seldom high enough to stimulate much in the way of muscle growth, but the amount of training is so great that they remain in a constant run-down condition.

High-intensity exercise and a large amount of exercise are mutually exclusive factors. You can have one or the other, but not both at the same time.

Get serious. Make all your exercise intense. But keep it brief.

On each exercise, do all the repetitions you possibly can...and then try one more!

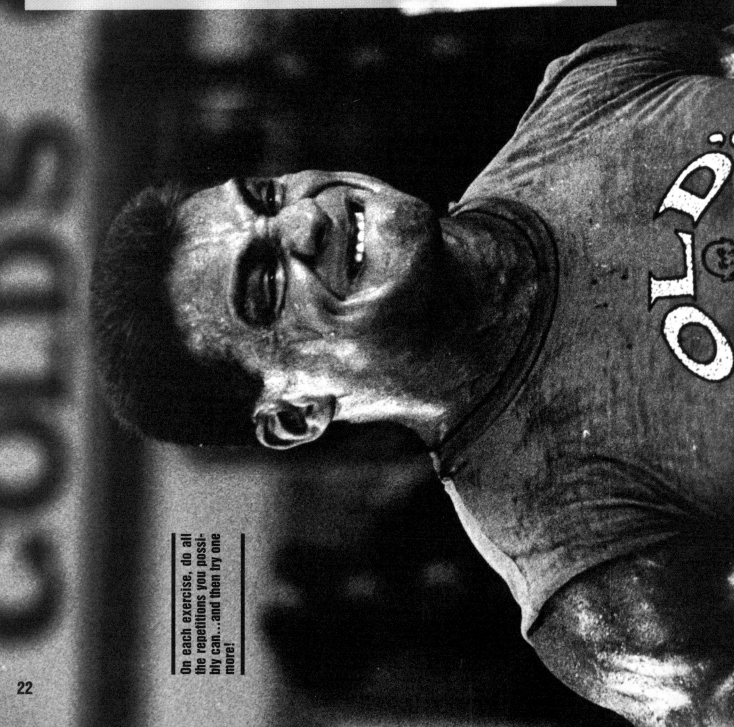

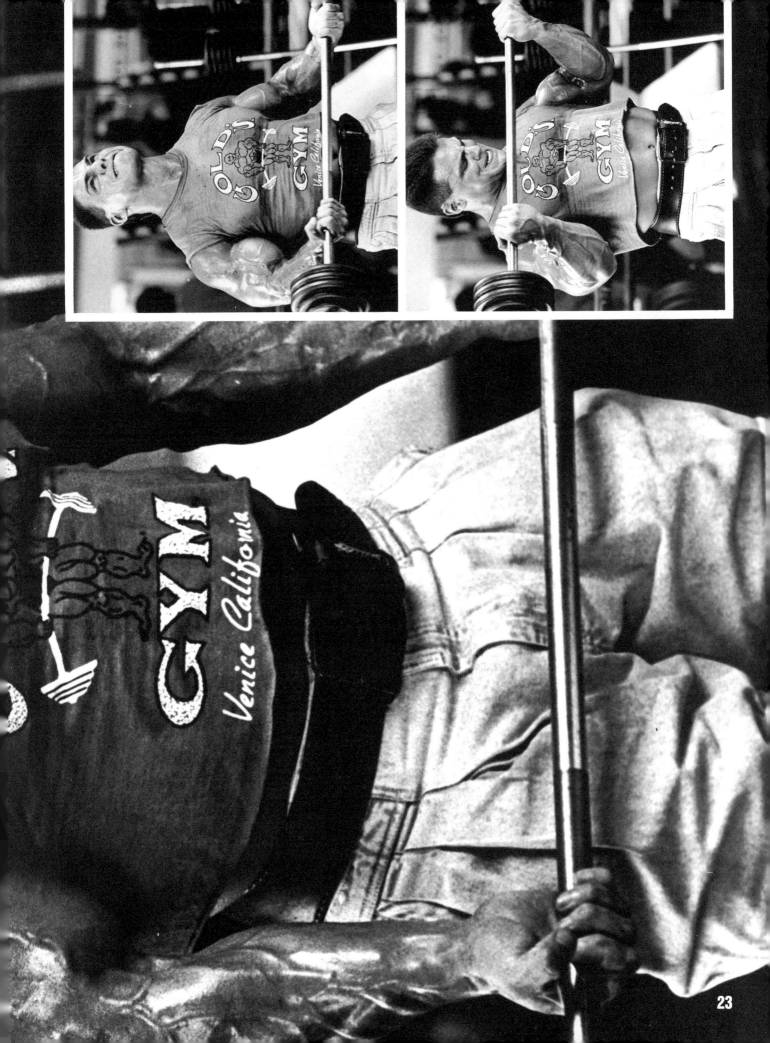

23

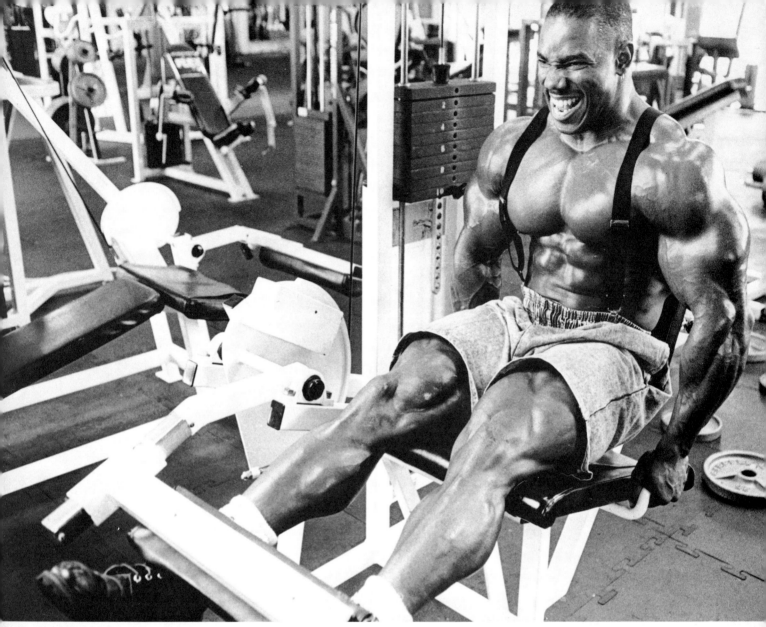

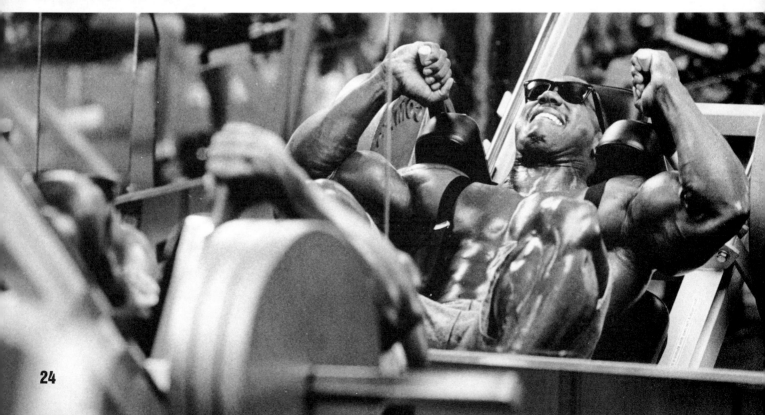

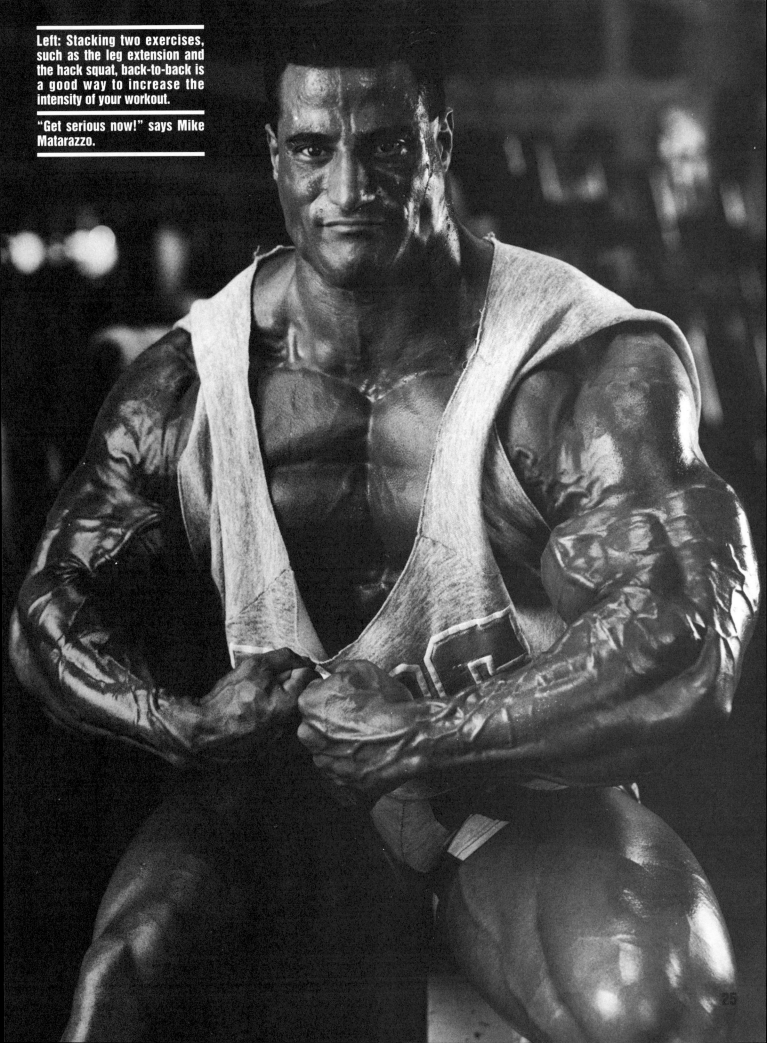

Left: Stacking two exercises, such as the leg extension and the hack squat, back-to-back is a good way to increase the intensity of your workout.

"Get serious now!" says Mike Matarazzo.

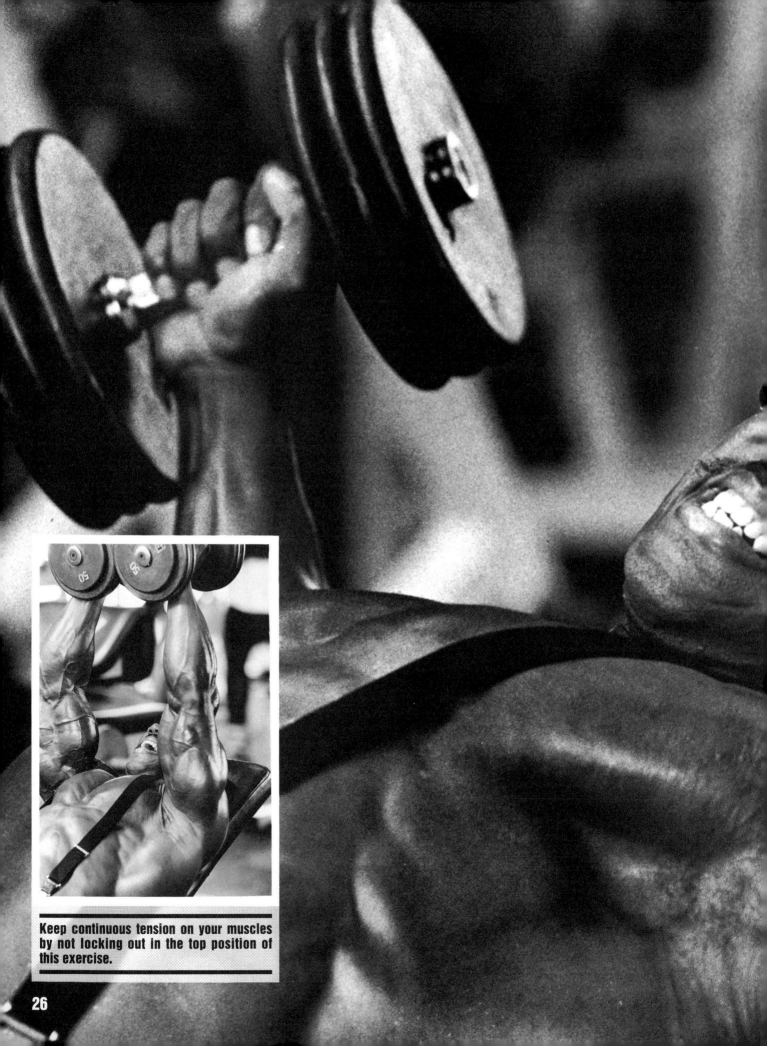

Keep continuous tension on your muscles by not locking out in the top position of this exercise.

5 • FORM

Your form in lifting and lowering the resistance is a key factor in the growth process. Form has a paradoxical influence on your response to exercise. Poor form is associated with a higher rate of performance improvement but a lower rate of muscle gain. For example, by training in a fast, momentum-assisted manner you can lift heavier weights. But because more momentum means less muscle tension, your performance increases will be much greater than your growth increases.

Poor form brings surrounding muscle groups into action to initiate and assist the lifting movements. Slow, smooth exercise form facilitates muscle isolation and intensity. Slow movements reduce your momentum, and, as a result, you lift less weight. However, the targeted muscle groups are fully responsible for lifting and lowering the resistance. Thus, greater growth stimulation is produced.

How slow should you move on each repetition? The rate advocated in this book is approximately four seconds on the positive phase and four seconds on the negative. That's four seconds up and four seconds down, or eight seconds per repetition. Naturally, long-range exercises will require more time than short-range movements.

The important concept to remember is to keep the momentum out of your exercise. This is best accomplished by strict, slow, smooth repetitions.

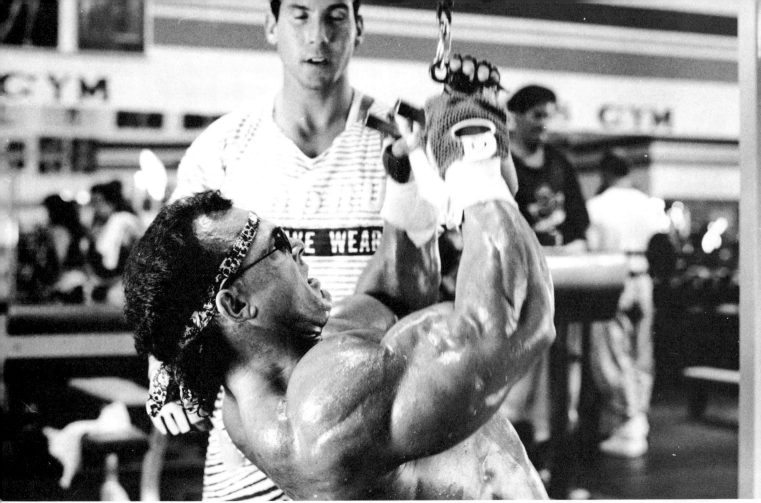

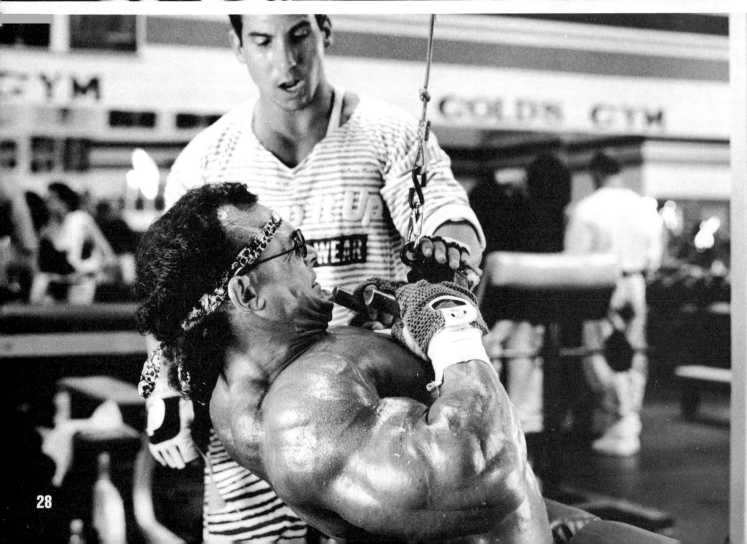

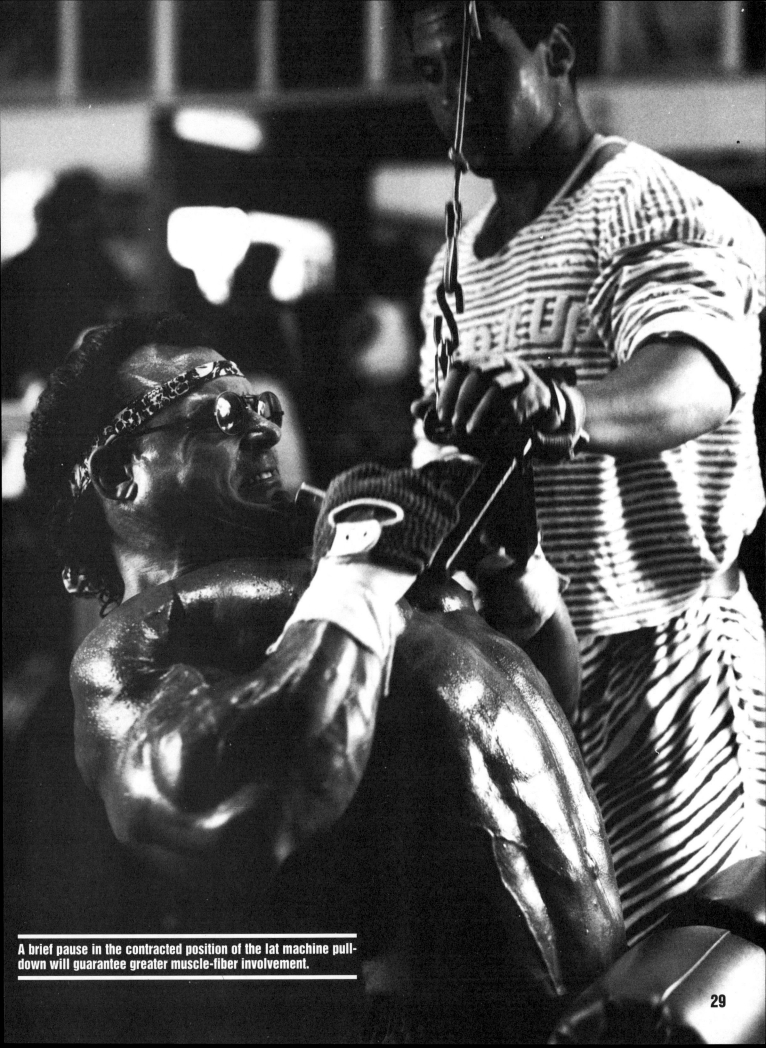

A brief pause in the contracted position of the lat machine pulldown will guarantee greater muscle-fiber involvement.

6 • REPETITIONS

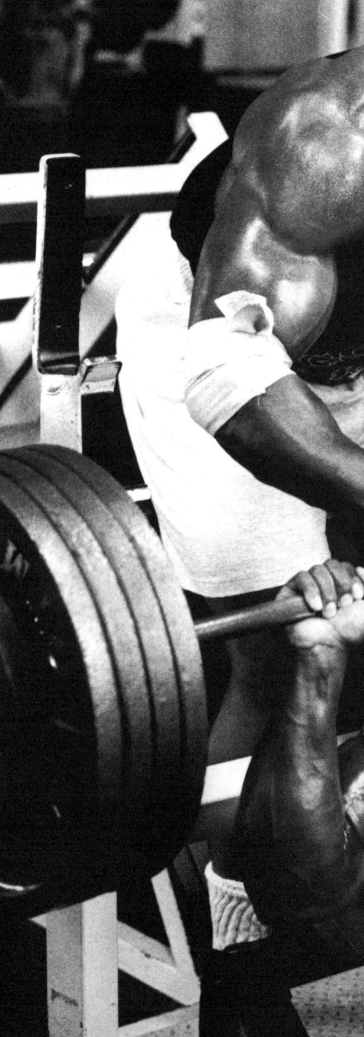

How many repetitions should you do for maximum muscle growth?

Repetitions are actually not as important as the amount of time a muscle spends under continuous tension. For best results, momentary muscular fatigue of the involved muscles should occur in 30 to 90 seconds.

Using the slow lifting and lowering form described in Chapter 5, most bodybuilders can perform 4 to 5 repetitions in 30 seconds, 8 to 10 in 60 seconds, and 12 to 15 in 90 seconds. Thus, the popular repetition scheme of 8 to 12 is effective for most trainees. I recommend 8 to 12 repetitions initially for all people I train.

Some bodybuilders find they get better results from slightly lower or higher repetition schemes. If you've been training for at least six months, you should already know the plan that works best for your body.

Regardless of the repetition guidelines you use, make certain that you fatigue each muscle in 30 to 90 seconds. Also, make sure that you do not simply stop an exercise because you've completed a specific amount of time or a repetition number. Always try one more repetition even when it seems impossible. Try continually to increase your intensity.

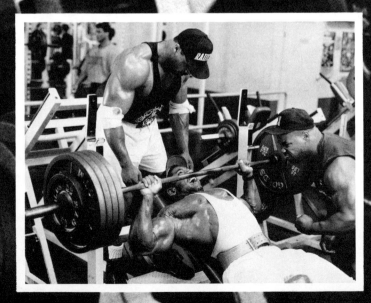

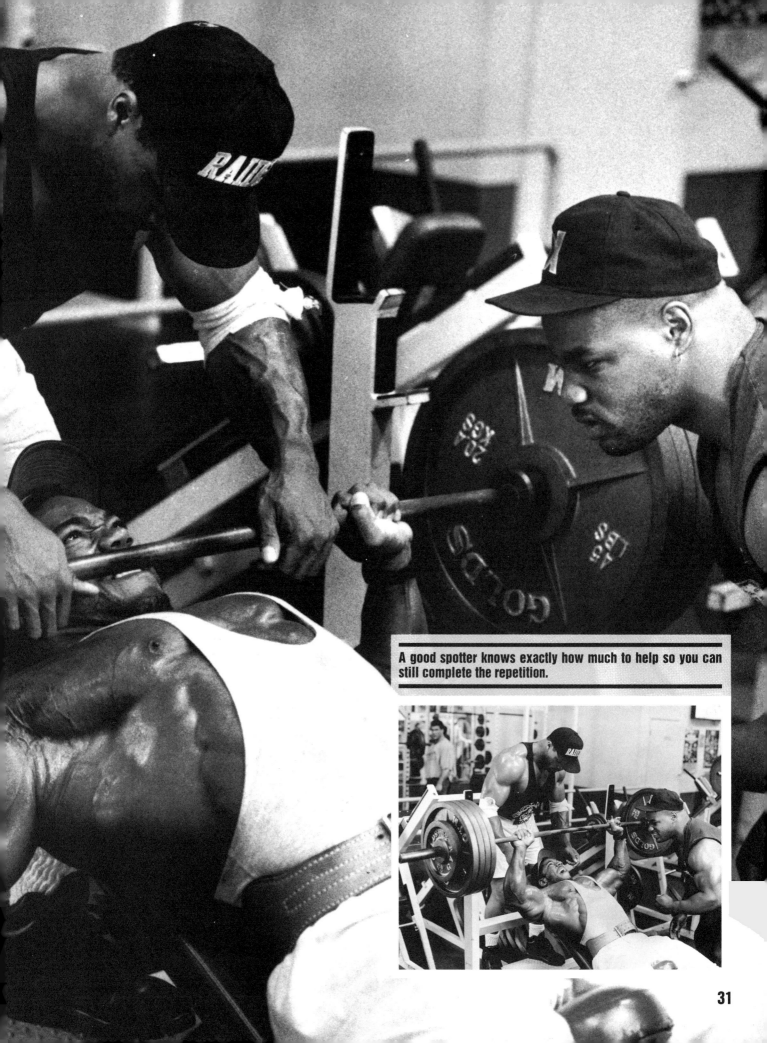

A good spotter knows exactly how much to help so you can still complete the repetition.

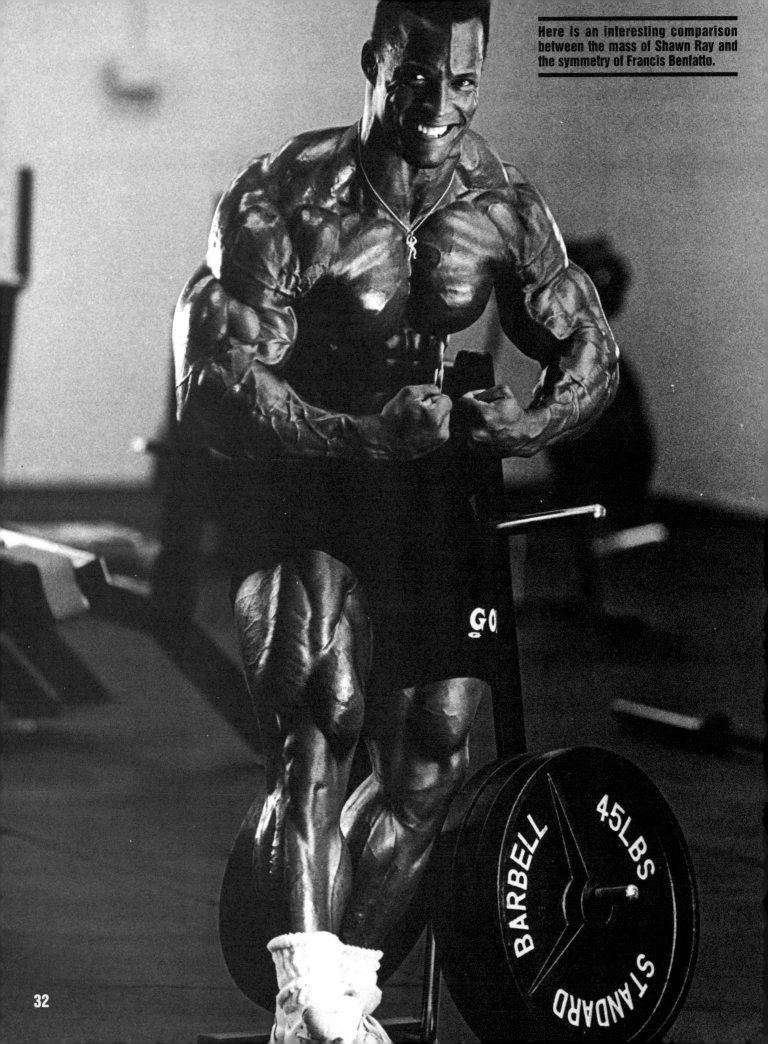

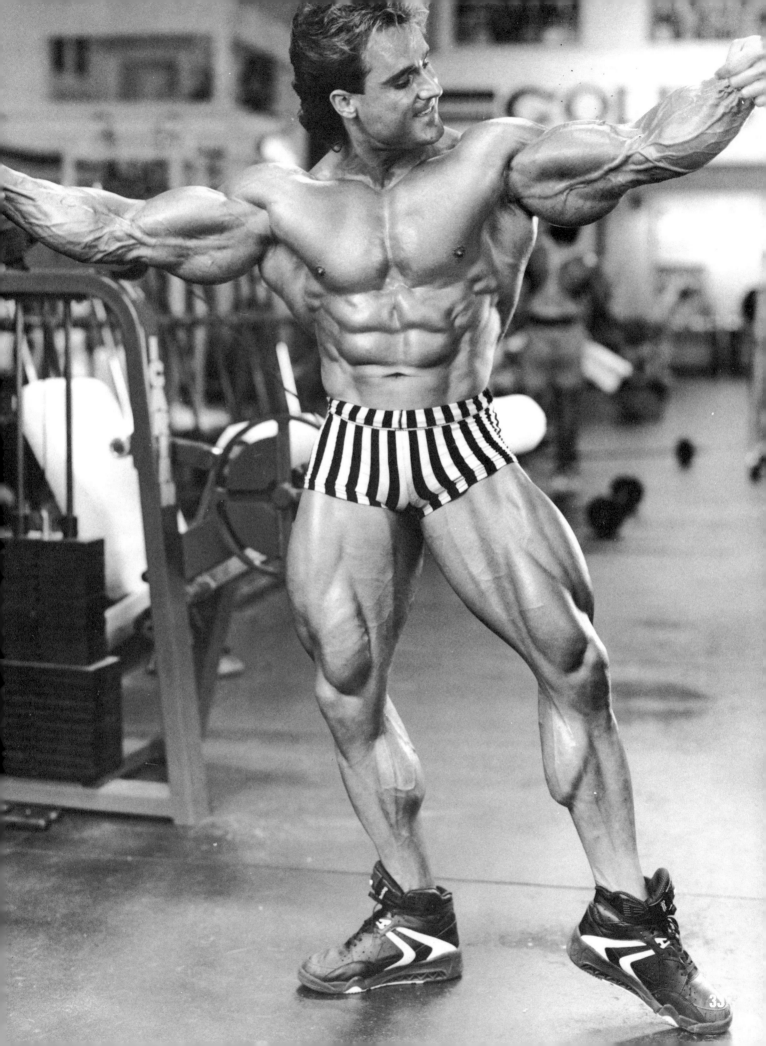

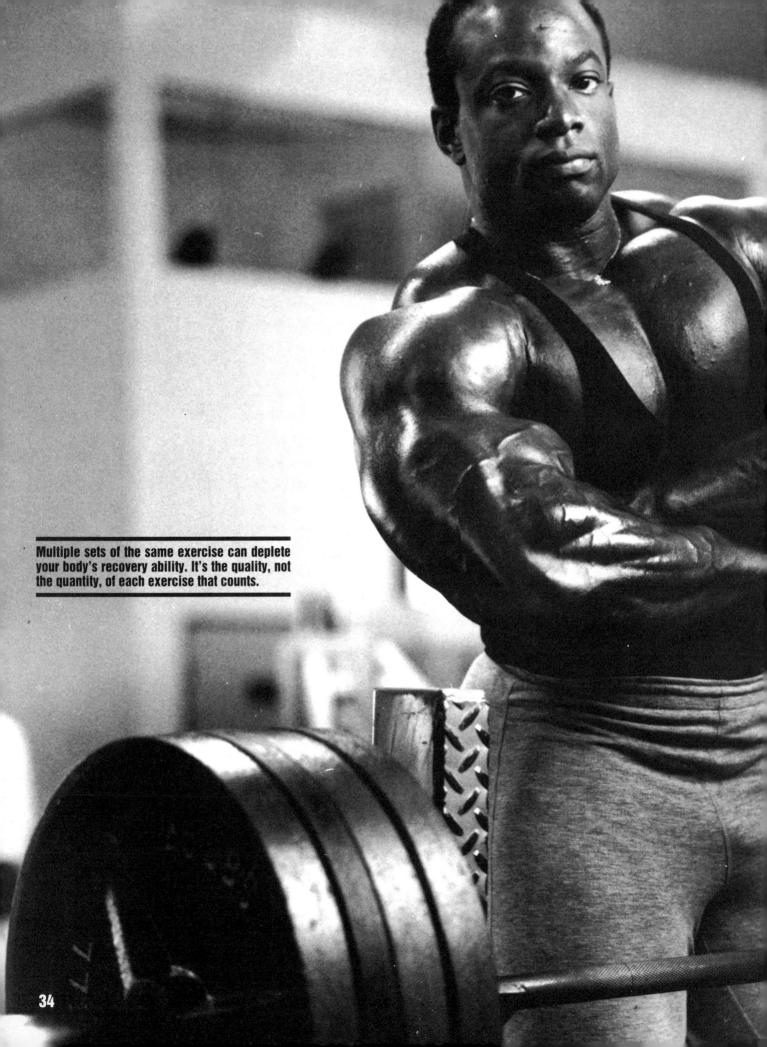

Multiple sets of the same exercise can deplete your body's recovery ability. It's the quality, not the quantity, of each exercise that counts.

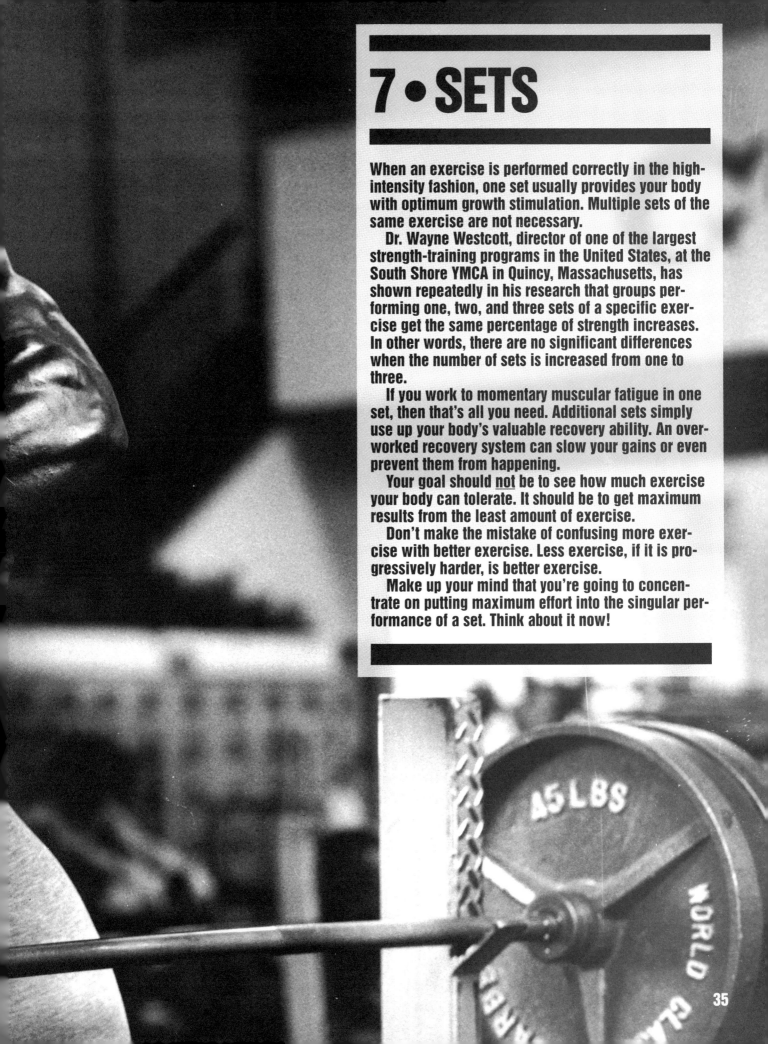

7 • SETS

When an exercise is performed correctly in the high-intensity fashion, one set usually provides your body with optimum growth stimulation. Multiple sets of the same exercise are not necessary.

Dr. Wayne Westcott, director of one of the largest strength-training programs in the United States, at the South Shore YMCA in Quincy, Massachusetts, has shown repeatedly in his research that groups performing one, two, and three sets of a specific exercise get the same percentage of strength increases. In other words, there are no significant differences when the number of sets is increased from one to three.

If you work to momentary muscular fatigue in one set, then that's all you need. Additional sets simply use up your body's valuable recovery ability. An overworked recovery system can slow your gains or even prevent them from happening.

Your goal should not be to see how much exercise your body can tolerate. It should be to get maximum results from the least amount of exercise.

Don't make the mistake of confusing more exercise with better exercise. Less exercise, if it is progressively harder, is better exercise.

Make up your mind that you're going to concentrate on putting maximum effort into the singular performance of a set. Think about it now!

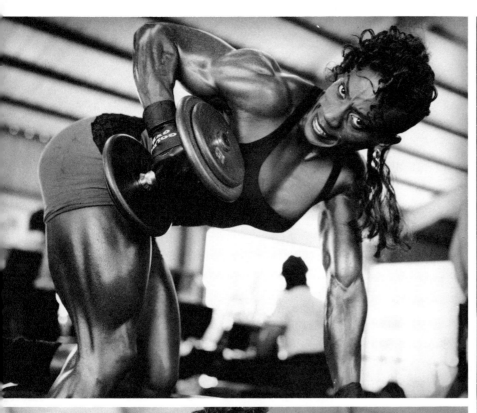

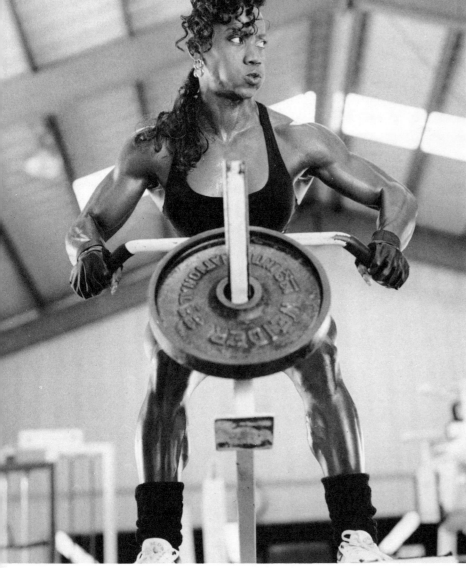

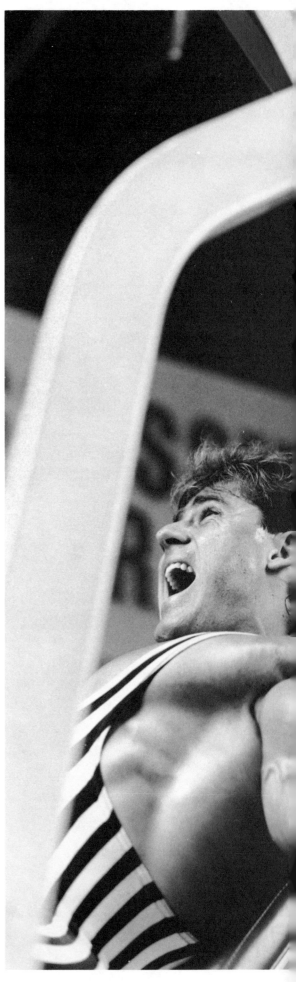

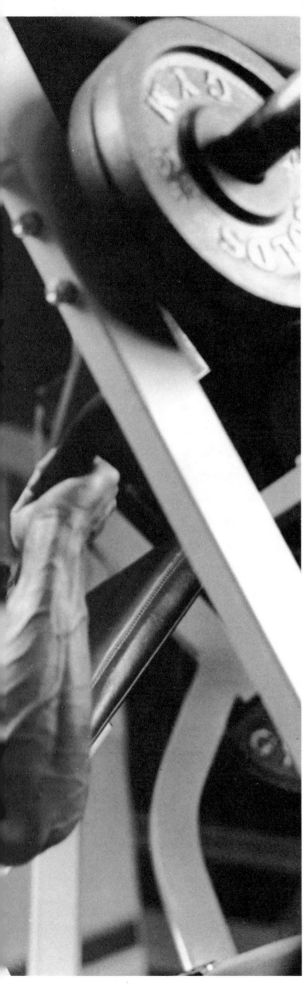

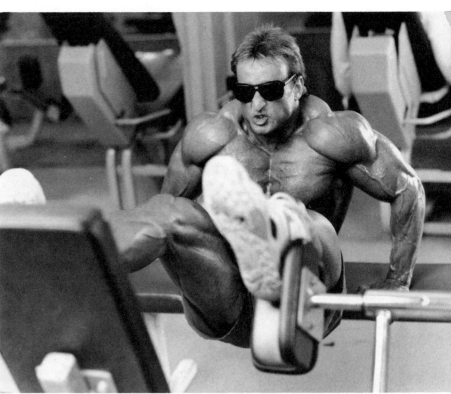

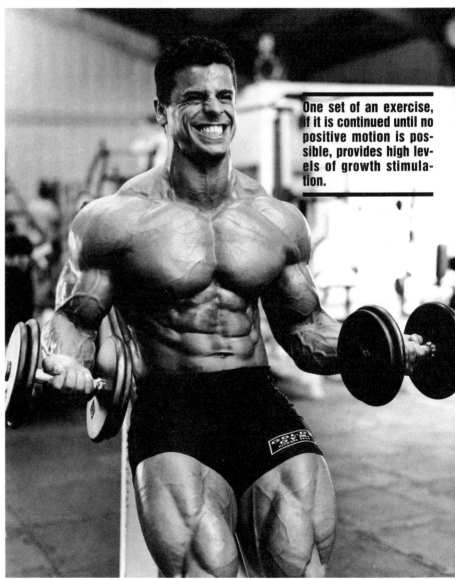

One set of an exercise, if it is continued until no positive motion is possible, provides high levels of growth stimulation.

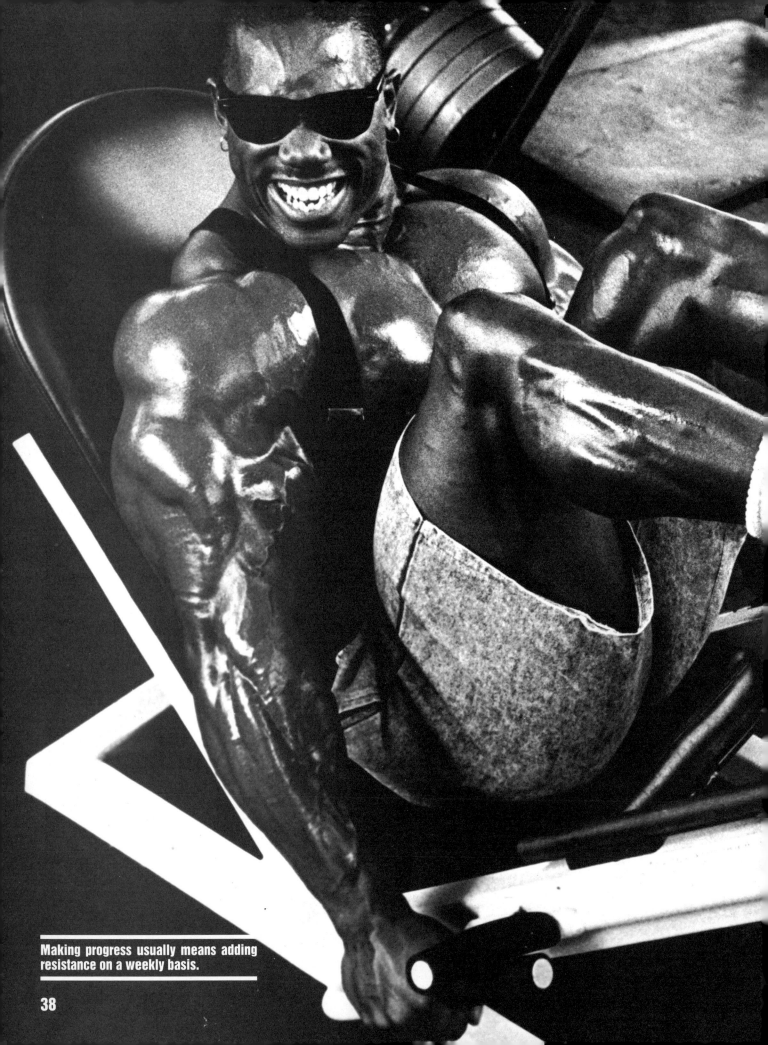

Making progress usually means adding resistance on a weekly basis.

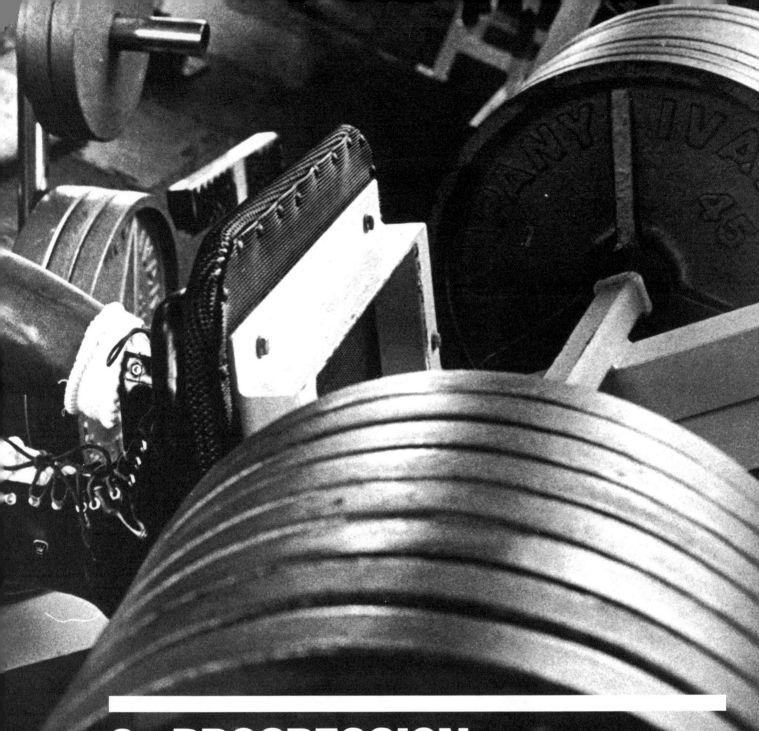

8 • PROGRESSION

You should make progress in each workout. Progress is achieved by increasing the repetitions or resistance in each exercise.

If you are performing between 8 and 12 repetitions on all your exercises, for example, then being able to do 12 or more is a sign that you should increase the resistance at the next workout by approximately 5 percent. Doing so will reduce your repetitions to 8 or 9.

A 5 percent increase in resistance on each exercise per week will yield noticeable results within only a month.

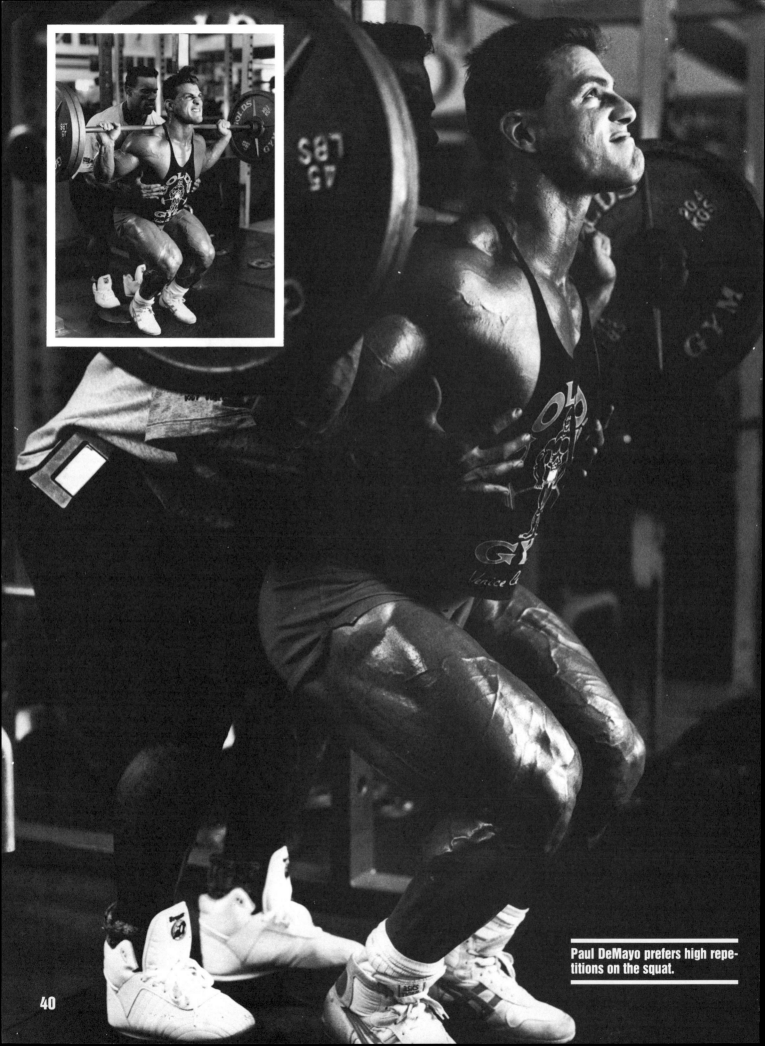

Paul DeMayo prefers high repetitions on the squat.

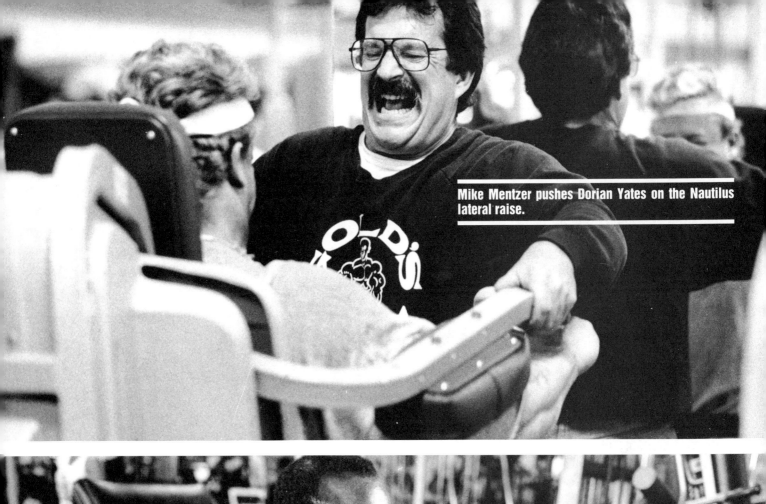

Mike Mentzer pushes Dorian Yates on the Nautilus lateral raise.

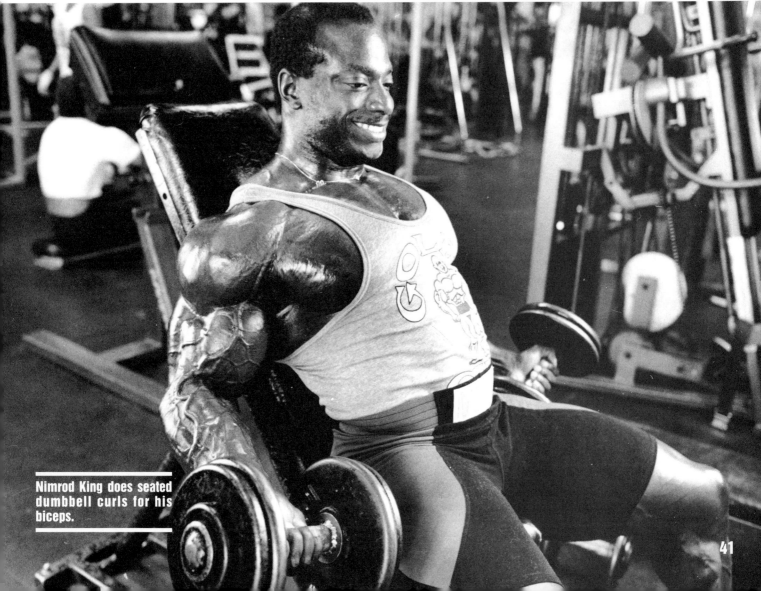

Nimrod King does seated dumbbell curls for his biceps.

9 • DURATION

How much time should you spend on each training session?

The various parts of your body usually are grouped into nine sections: hips, thighs, calves, shoulders, back, chest, arms, waist, and neck. Each of these body parts should be exercised at least two times per week. The total number of exercises per workout should vary from 10 to 20 depending on the equipment available.

Each exercise should be performed slowly for one set of 8 to 12 repetitions, or from 30 to 90 seconds, with approximately 60 seconds being the average time. No more than 60 seconds should elapse between exercises. A typical workout, therefore, should require between 25 and 45 minutes. None of the workouts described in Part IV took more than 30 minutes to complete.

It's to your advantage to look for ways to make your exercise harder and briefer. As a result your body will recover more completely and grow faster.

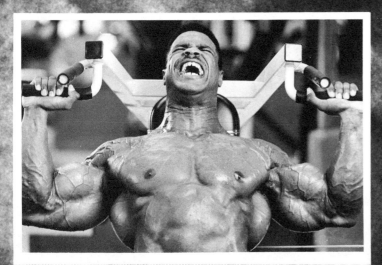

HUGE is the only way to describe Paul Dillett's arms!

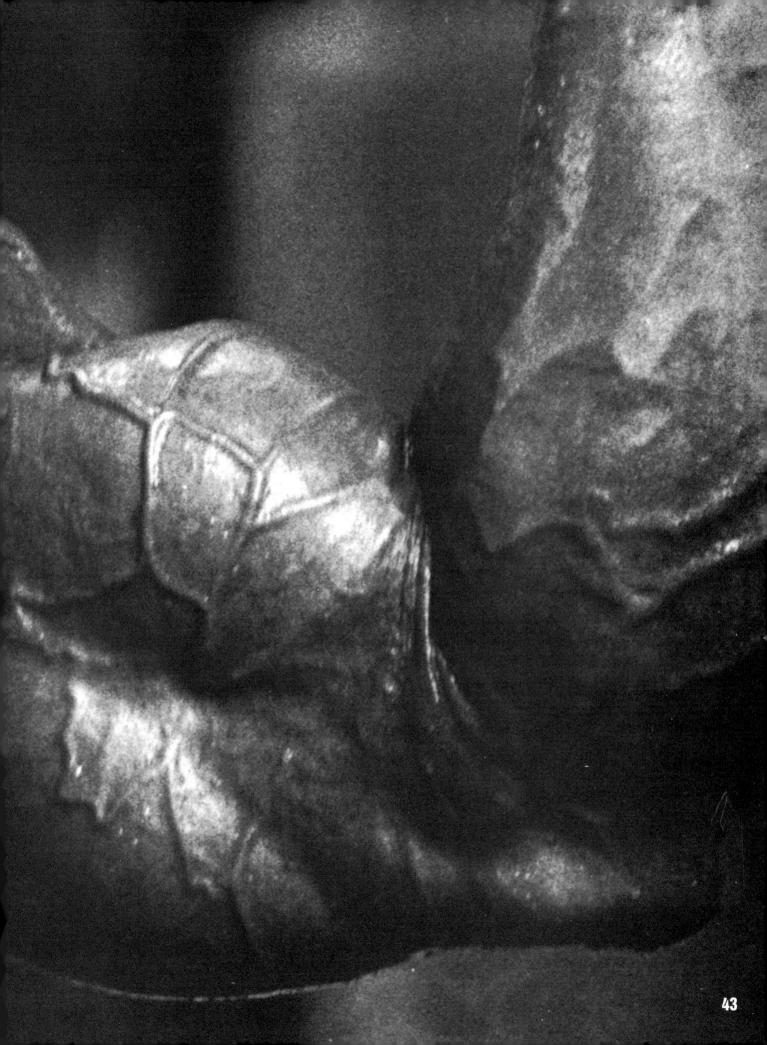

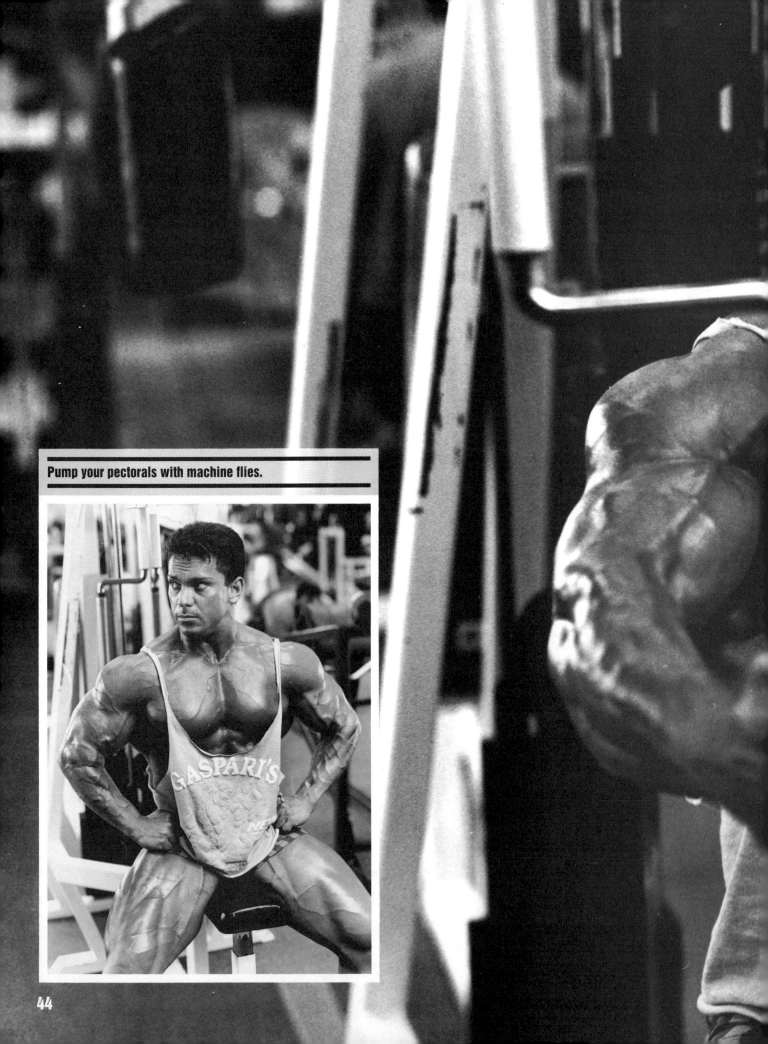

Pump your pectorals with machine flies.

SPARI'S
NEW AGE

FITNESS CENTER
OCEAN TWP. N.J. 07712

10 • FREQUENCY

Research shows that a seven-day cycle of training is nearly perfect for overall muscle growth. This is the case because it provides needed rest, recovery, and irregularity of training.

Your workouts proceed on Monday, Wednesday, and Friday. On Sunday your body is anticipating a workout but it doesn't come. Instead, it occurs the next day when your body is not expecting it.

With almost 48 hours of rest between two workouts and almost 72 hours after the third, a three-times-per-week exercise schedule allows for consistent growth stimulation and recovery overcompensation within your major muscle groups.

Best results usually occur when you do <u>not</u> split your routine into upper body one day and lower body the next day. Split routines lead to overtraining.

A total body routine that is repeated three times per week is best for short-term and long-term growth.

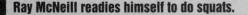

Ray McNeill readies himself to do squats.

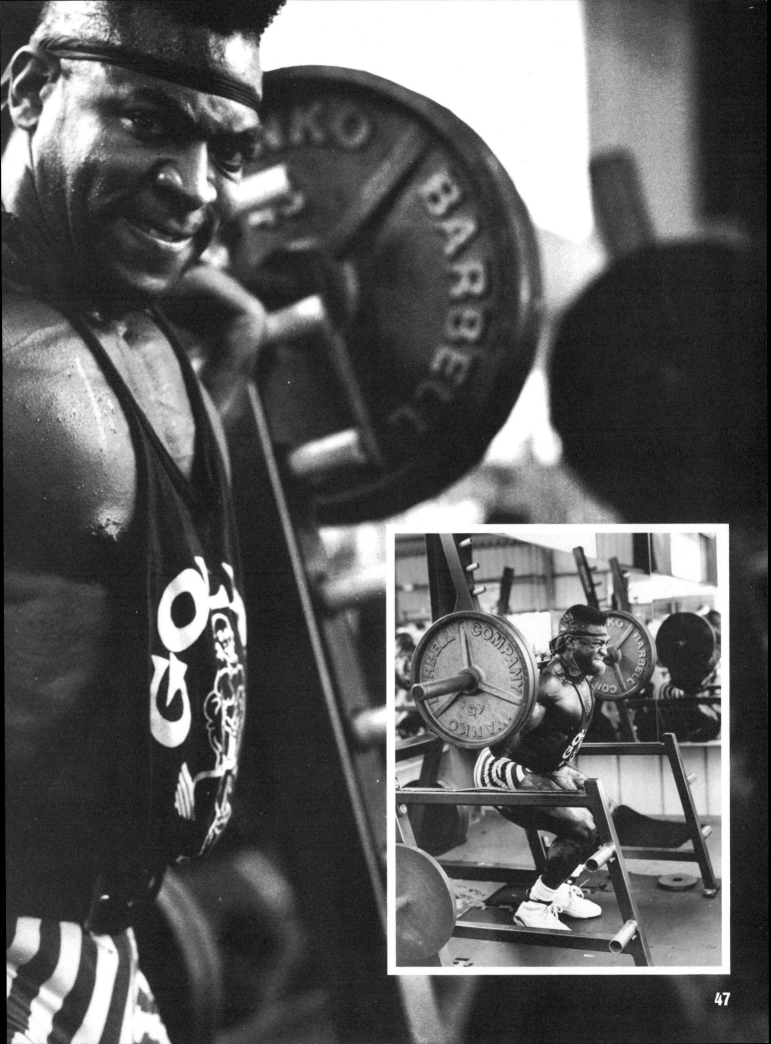

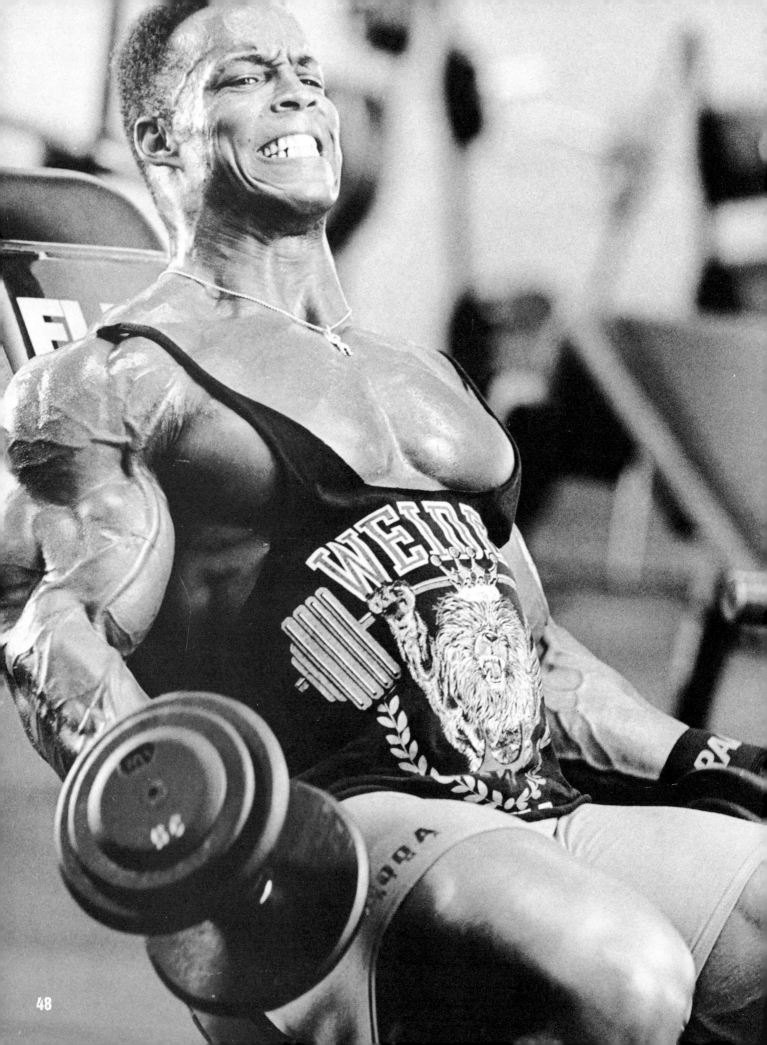

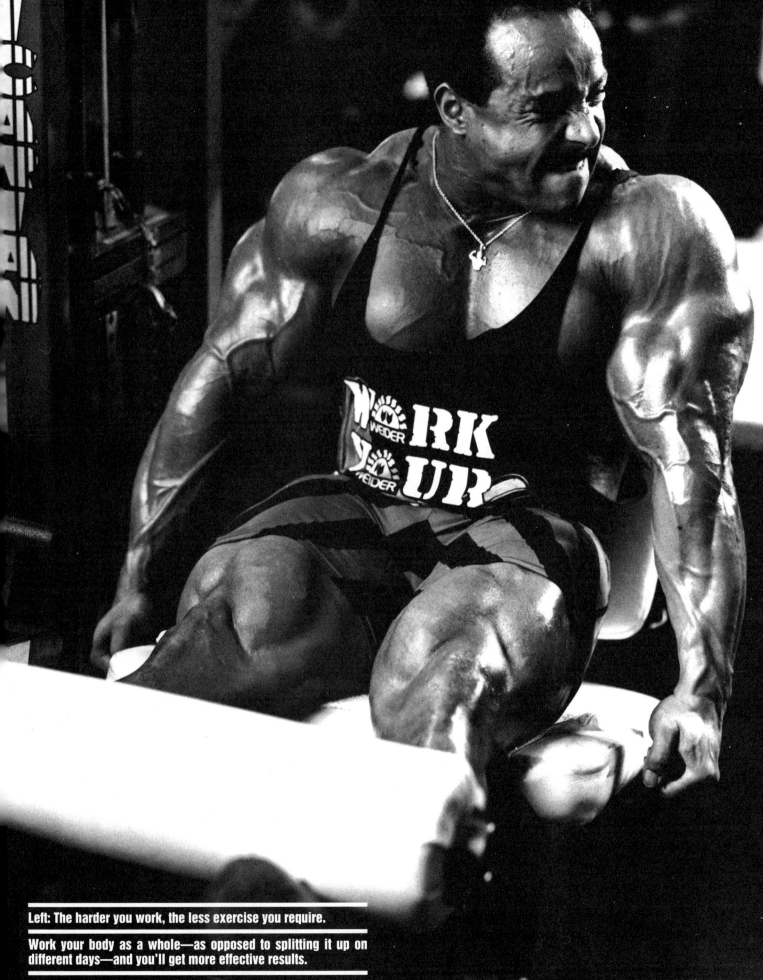

Left: The harder you work, the less exercise you require.

Work your body as a whole—as opposed to splitting it up on different days—and you'll get more effective results.

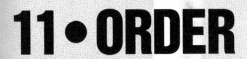

11 • ORDER

You'll get better overall growth stimulation if your muscles are worked in the order of their relative sizes, from largest to smallest.

This means that usually you should work your lower body before your upper body. This, for example, would be an acceptable order: hips, thighs, calves, shoulders, back, chest, arms, waist, and neck.

Exceptions to this guideline would include specialized routines where you emphasize certain body parts, such as the arms or chest. In these cases, you'd work your arms or chest first and then follow the normal order of the routine minus the specialized body part.

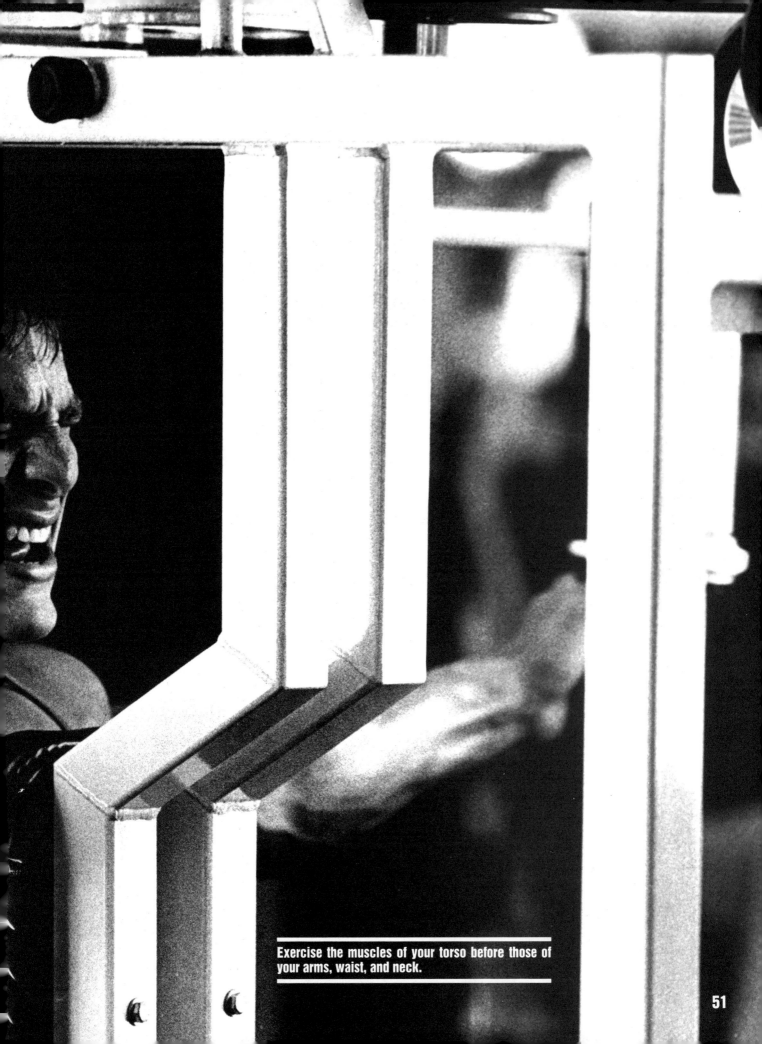

Exercise the muscles of your torso before those of your arms, waist, and neck.

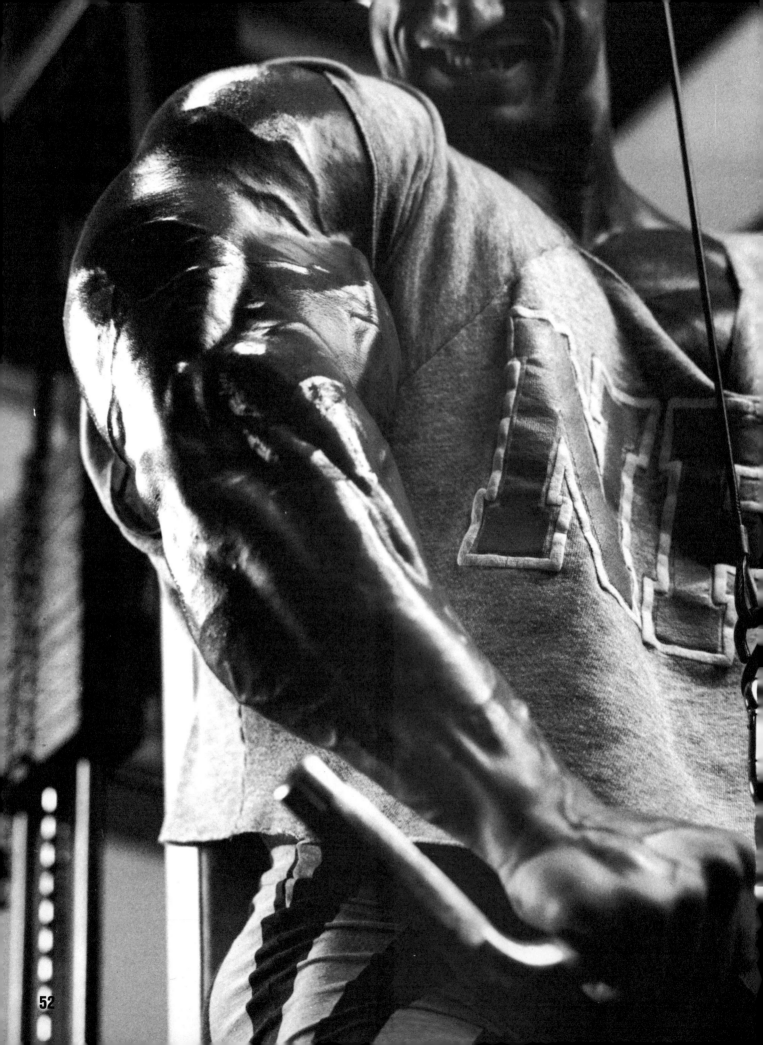

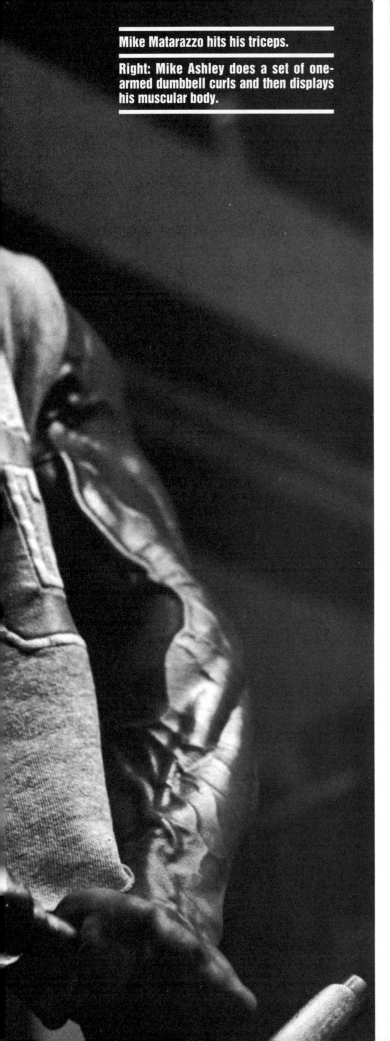

Mike Matarazzo hits his triceps.

Right: Mike Ashley does a set of one-armed dumbbell curls and then displays his muscular body.

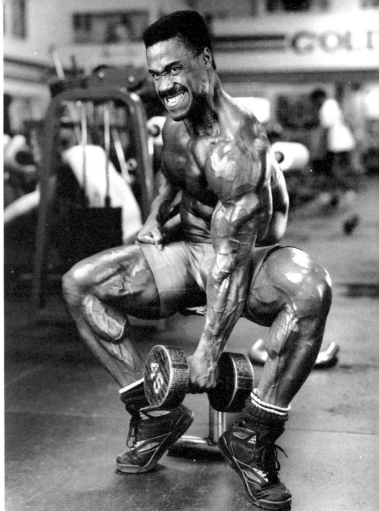

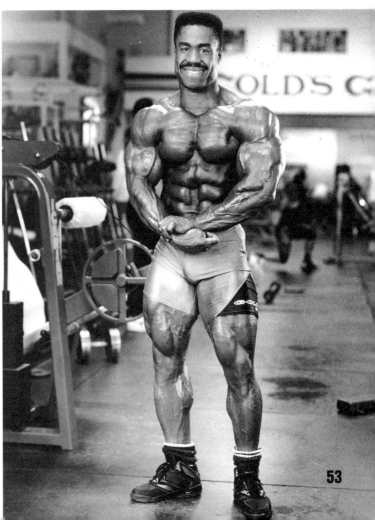

53

12 • VARIETY

Certain exercise variations can keep you from getting bored. Three special techniques—pre-exhaustion sets, negative-only training, and the 1½-repetition chin-up and dip—will be discussed fully in Part IV. Here is a brief description of each.

Pre-exhaustion sets involve stacking two or three exercises for the same body part back-to-back. Usually a single-joint movement for a specific muscle is immediately followed by a related multiple-joint exercise. Or you can do a multiple-joint movement, a single-joint exercise, and then another multiple-joint movement.

Negative-only training takes advantage of the fact that you are 40 percent stronger lowering a weight than you are raising it. To utilize negative-only training, you'll need a partner to help you lift the barbell or machine's movement arm to the top or contracted position. After a smooth transfer, lower the resistance very slowly back to the starting position.

Or you can do negative-only chins and dips unassisted by using your legs to climb to the top position. Then lower yourself very slowly.

The 1½-repetition chin-up or dip is performed by starting at the top. Take a slow 30 seconds to do the negative phase, another 30 seconds on the positive position, and a final 30 seconds on the negative part. This makes for a very difficult chin-up or dip.

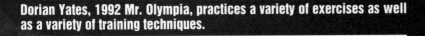

Dorian Yates, 1992 Mr. Olympia, practices a variety of exercises as well as a variety of training techniques.

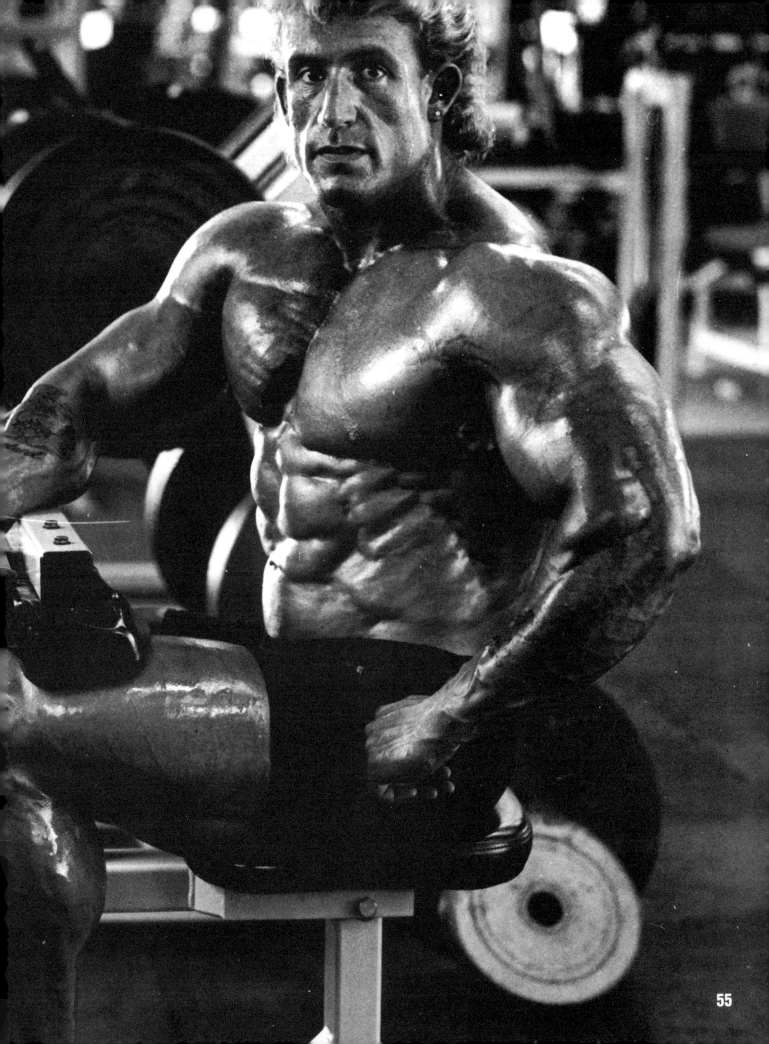

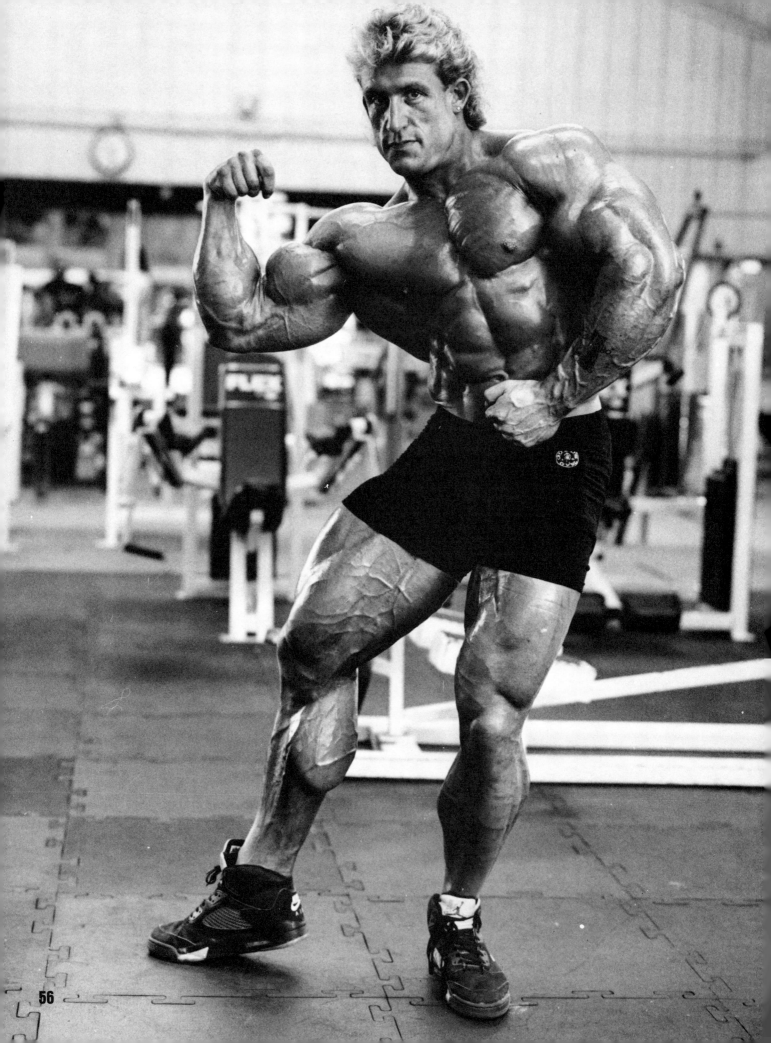

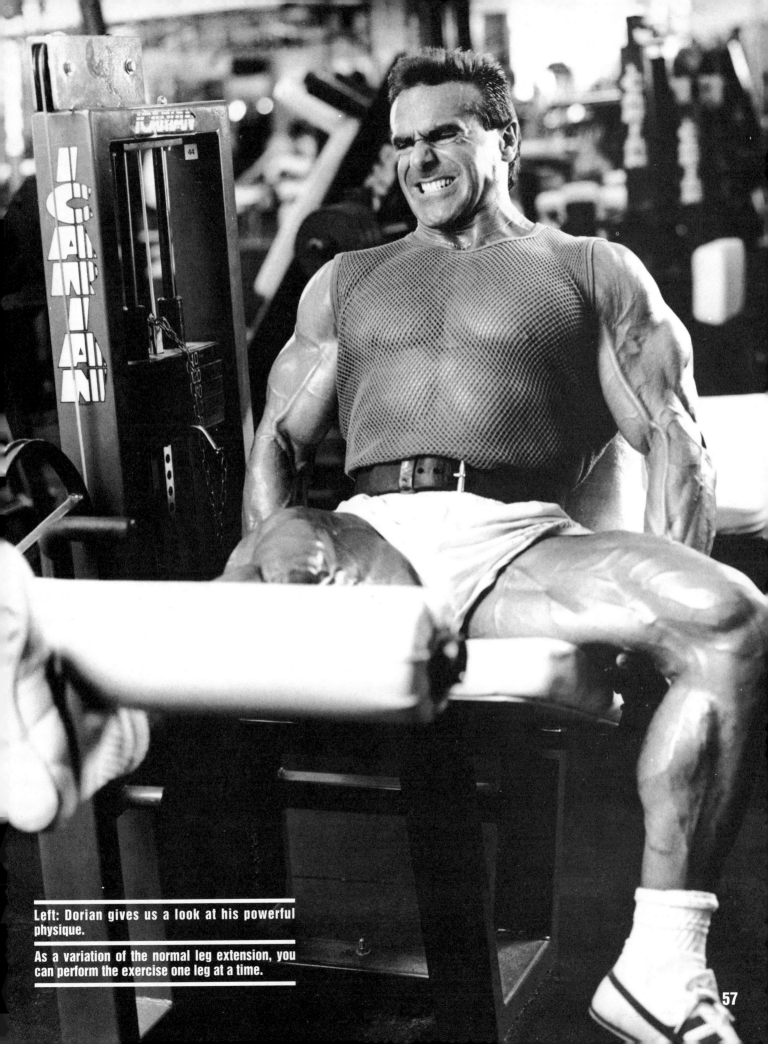

Left: Dorian gives us a look at his powerful physique.

As a variation of the normal leg extension, you can perform the exercise one leg at a time.

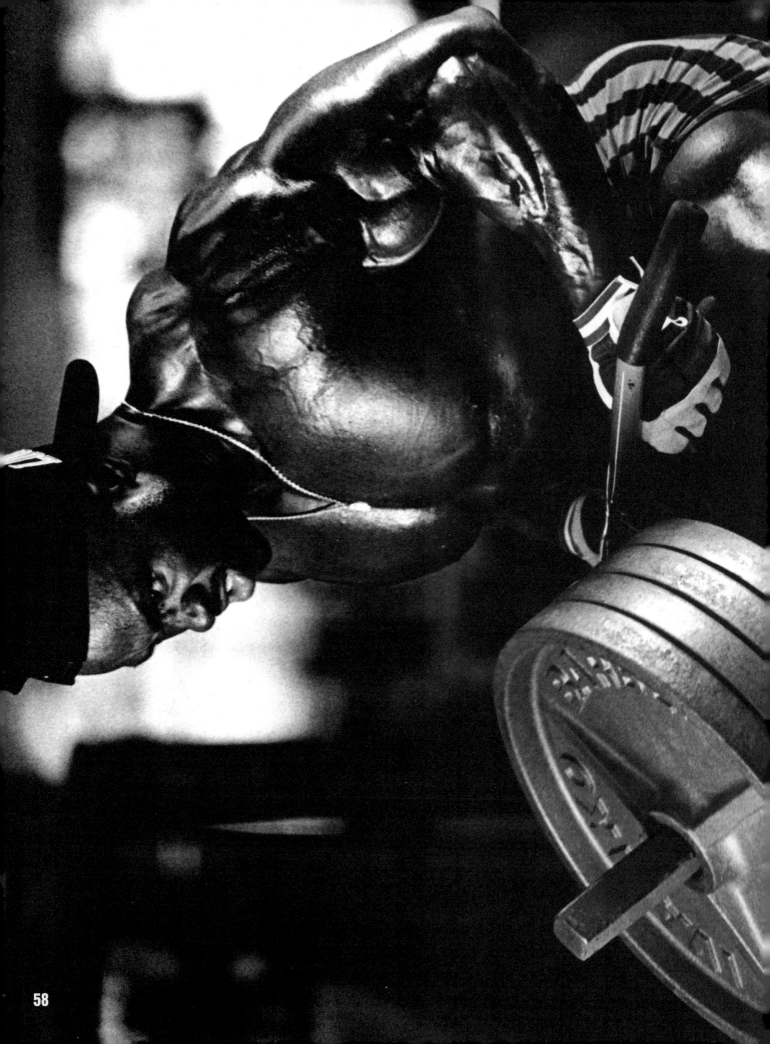

13.
WARM-UP

An elaborate warm-up is not necessary before your workout. In fact, each set of 8 to 12 repetitions includes a built-in warm-up: your initial 6 or 7 repetitions act as an effective warm-up for your last several repetitions, which are the hardest.

Competitive weightlifters, however, do need to do several sets of progressively heavier lifts before they attempt their maximums. Such warm-ups may also be psychologically beneficial to the lifter.

A muscular John Sherman works his upper body.

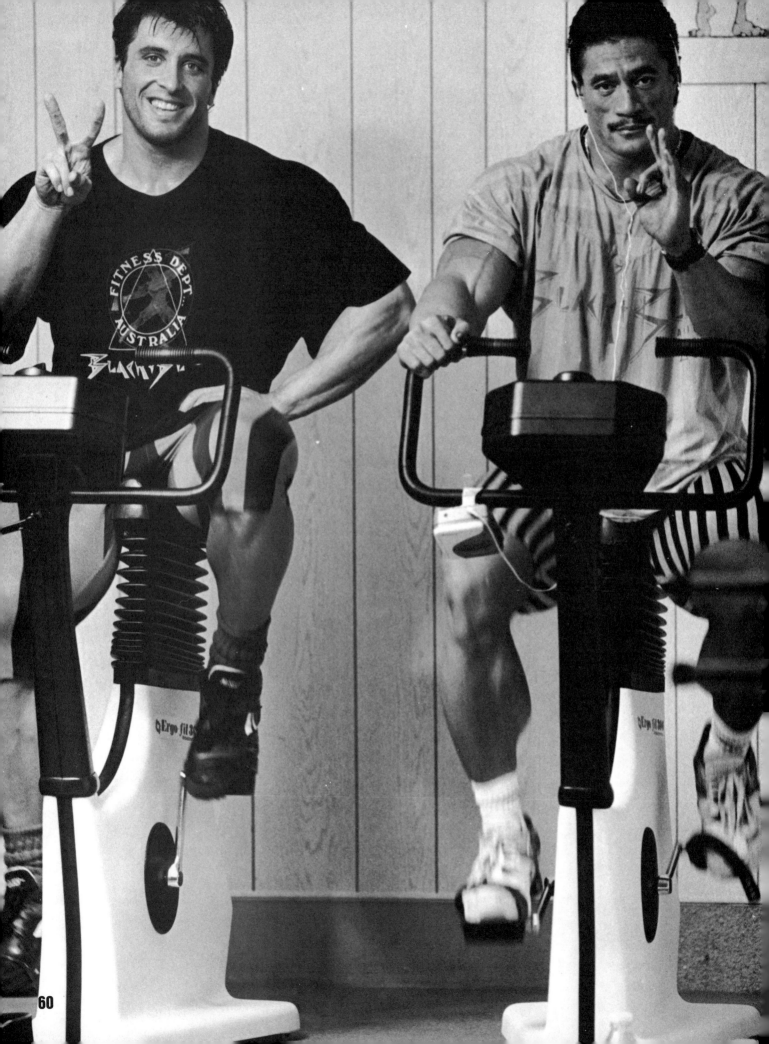

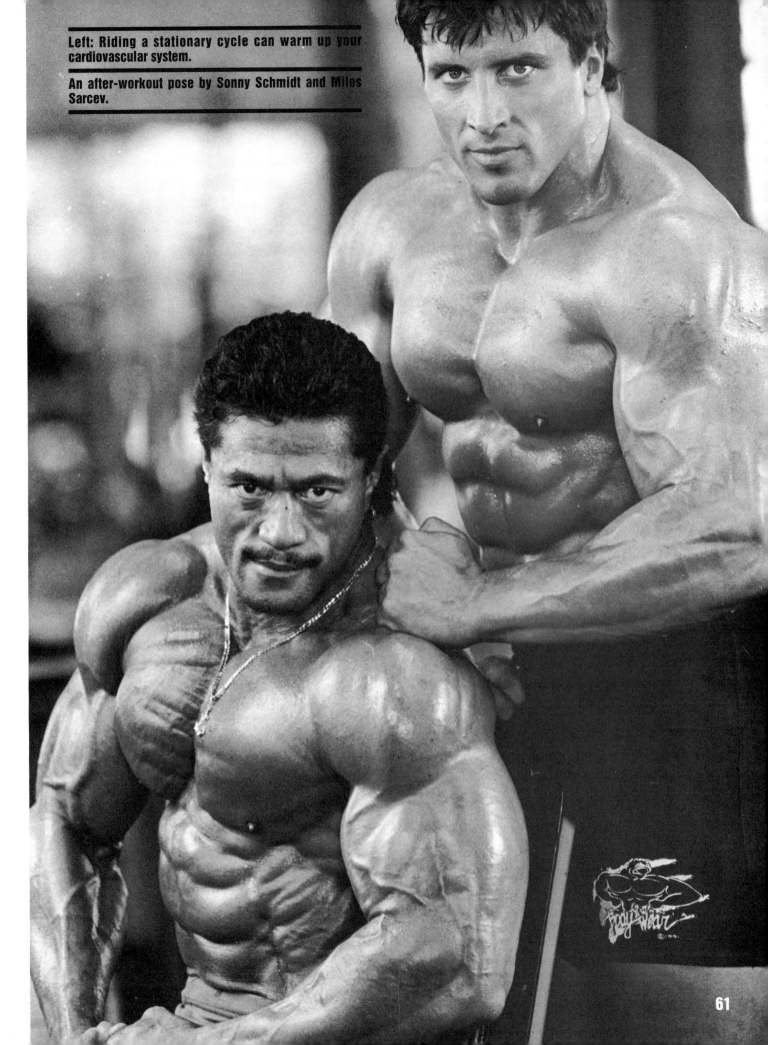

14 •
OVERTRAINING

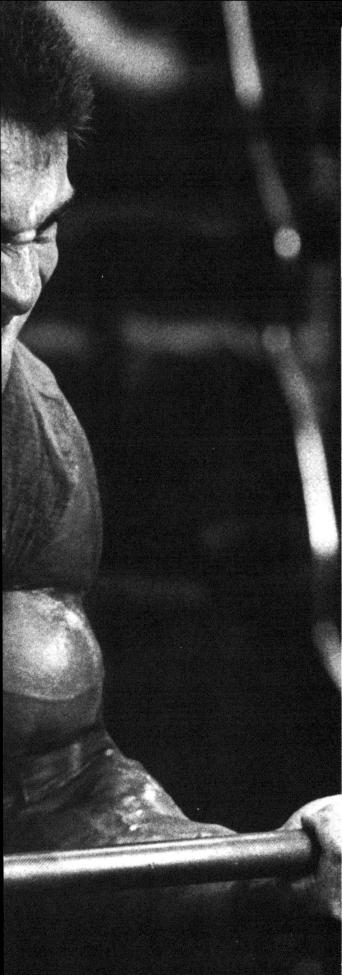

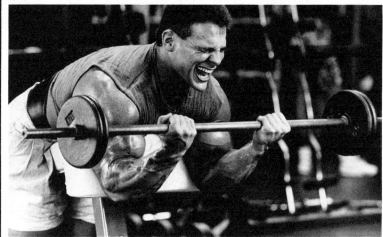

Most bodybuilders are addicted to long, multiple-set routines, which lead to overtraining.

Overtraining results from too much exercise and too little rest and recuperation. It leads to a reduction in muscular size, strength, and performance.

Proper exercise creates a need for growth. It makes demands on your body that cannot be met by your existing muscular development. But you must understand that exercise is only the stimulus. Once the stimulus is applied, you must back off and permit your body to respond—that is, to grow.

Unfortunately, it is difficult for most bodybuilders to retreat from their exercise. Overtraining is usually the result.

Here are the symptoms of overtraining:

- No training progress
- Decreased muscular size and strength
- Longer-than-average recovery time after a workout
- Increased heart rate during day off
- Increased blood pressure during day off
- Increased joint and muscle aches
- Loss of interest in training
- Lack of energy
- Headaches
- Hand tremors
- Loss or diminution of appetite
- Tiredness
- Irritability
- Listlessness
- Insomnia

As Arthur Jones, inventor of Nautilus equipment, summarized more than 20 years ago: "Best results will always be produced by the minimum amount of exercise that imposes the maximum amount of growth stimulation."

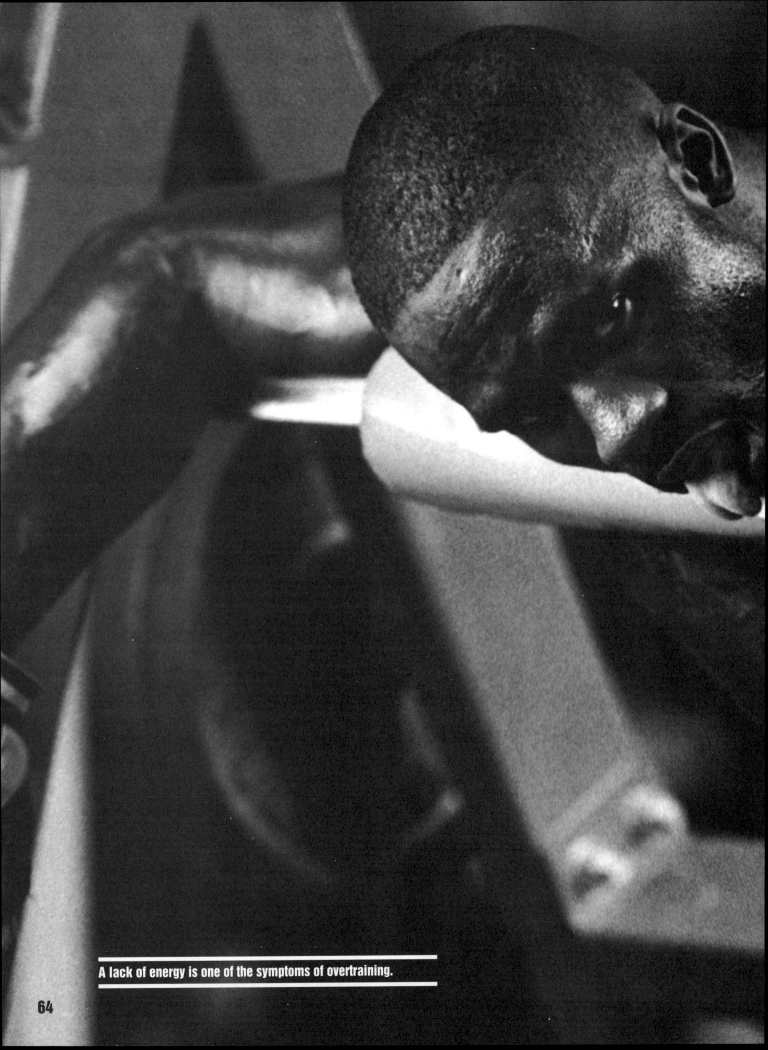

A lack of energy is one of the symptoms of overtraining.

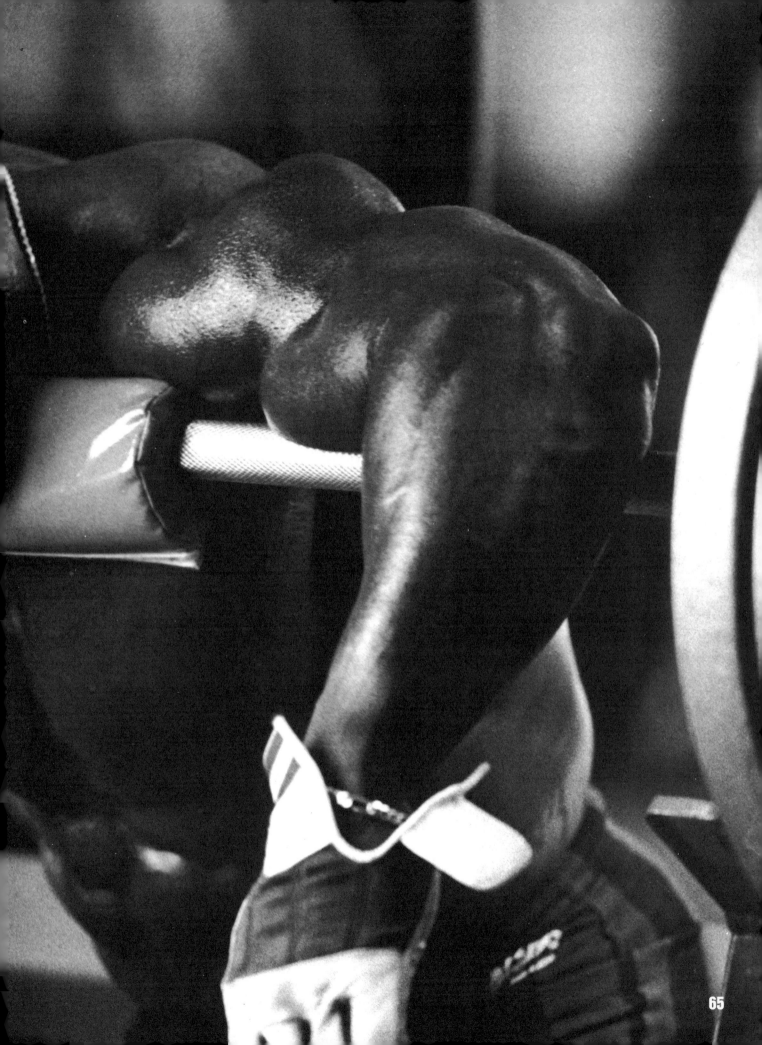

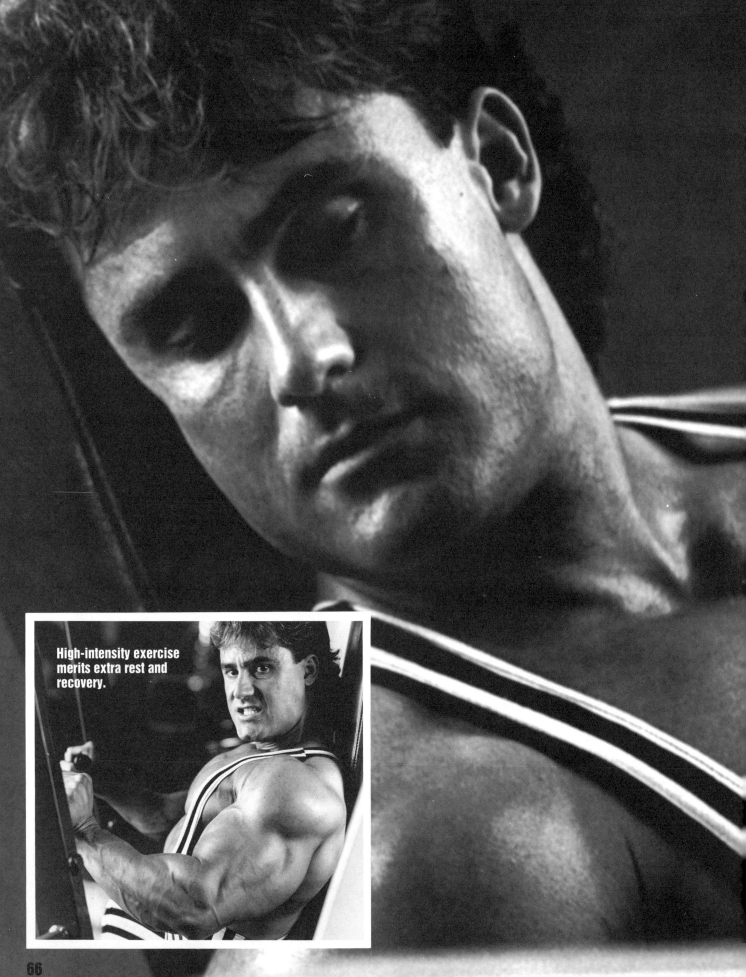

High-intensity exercise merits extra rest and recovery.

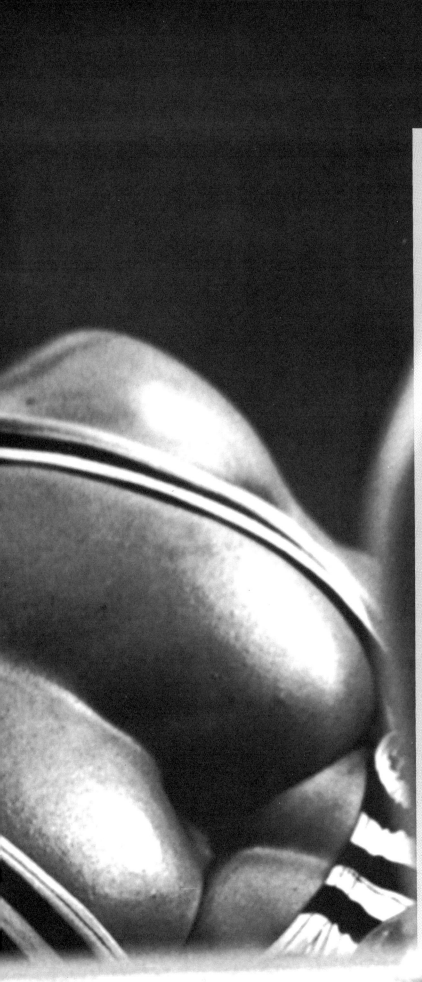

15 • REST

You must rest adequately if you want your muscles to grow. Research shows that actual muscle growth does not occur during exercising or eating but in resting situations, primarily while you are sleeping.

Newborn babies, for example, have phenomenal growth rates, and they sleep an average of 16 to 18 hours a day. By age one, 13 to 14 hours of daily sleep is the norm.

As children get older, their need for sleep gradually decreases until it levels off in adolescence. Teenagers usually require about 9½ hours of sleep per night.

Sleep time decreases again during adulthood. Most adults find they need about 8 hours of sleep, although approximately 10 percent require more or less than that.

Here are my sleep and rest recommendations for the 28-day growth program described in Part IV:

- Sleep 9 hours each night if you are an adult and 10 hours if you are a teenager.
- Wake up at the same time every morning. If you feel you require more sleep, go to bed earlier rather than sleeping later.
- Schedule a 15-minute nap during the middle of the afternoon, if possible.
- Do not participate in any type of vigorous activity—such as jogging, cycling, dancing, or racquetball—on your non-workout days.
- Get involved in several nonstrenuous hobbies, such as reading, listening to music, or woodworking.

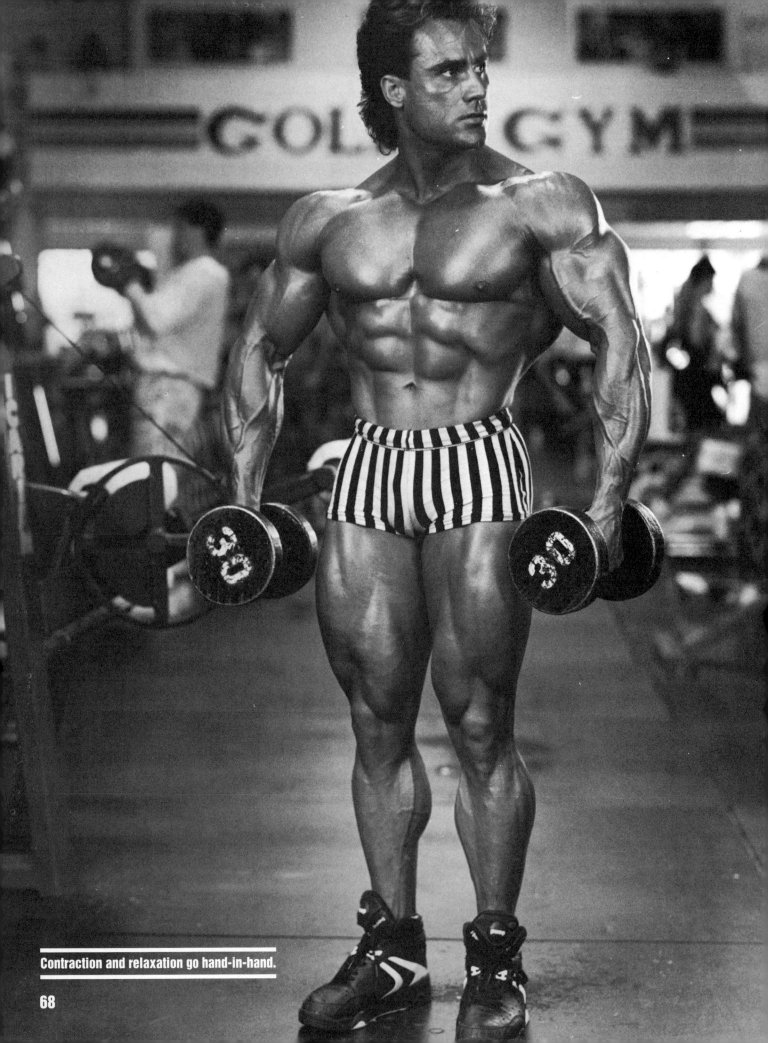

Contraction and relaxation go hand-in-hand.

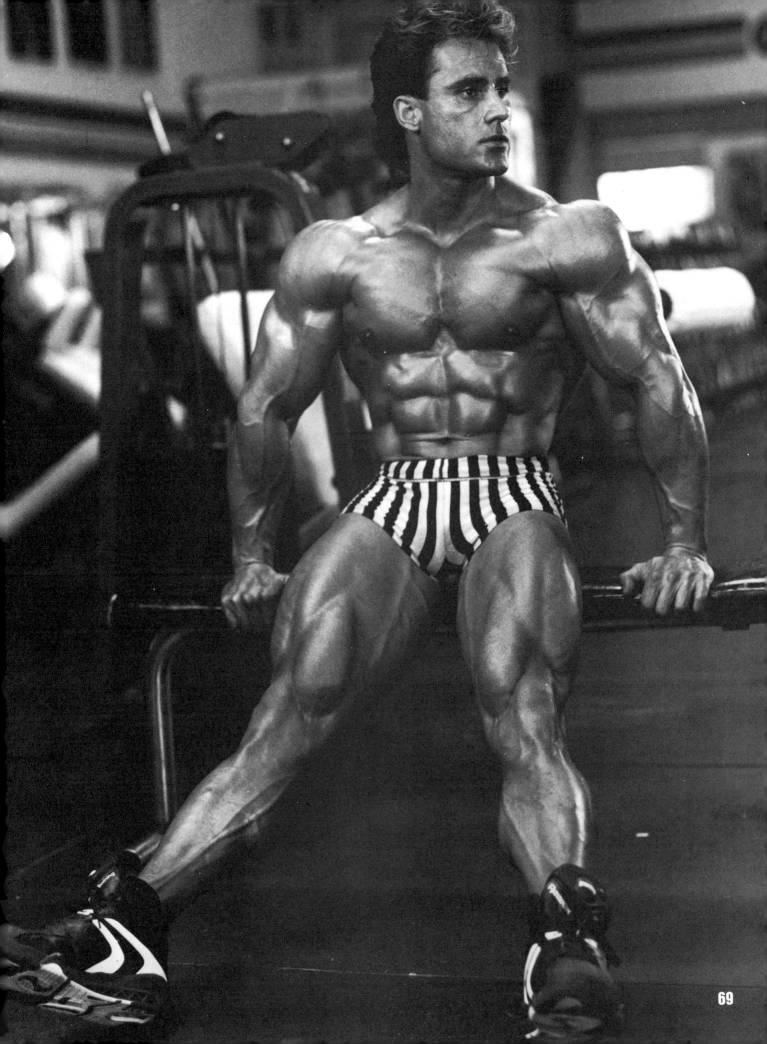

16 • POTENTIAL

Exercise increases the cross-sectional size of your muscles by adding the contractile proteins actin and myosin. There is little evidence that exercise increases the total number of muscle fibers. Greater muscle size results from enlargement, not proliferation, of individual muscle fibers.

The most important factor in your potential muscle size is the length of the muscle belly. The muscle belly represents the distance between the tendon attachments. The greater the distance, the greater the cross-sectional size and volume your muscles can be. Furthermore, the length of your muscle bellies is inherited and not subject to change through training.

Most people have muscle bellies throughout their bodies that are average in length. Some have a mixture of long, average, and short muscle bellies. A few have mostly short muscles, and very few have mostly long muscles. Long muscle bellies are a distinct advantage in growing larger and stronger.

Here are some examples of bodybuilders with long muscle bellies in certain body parts:

Biceps:	Mike Matarazzo, Vince Taylor, Paul Dillett
Triceps:	Thierry Pastel, Shawn Ray, Kevin Levrone
Quadriceps:	Paul DeMayo, Kevin Levrone
Hamstrings:	Shawn Ray, Paul DeMayo
Latissimus dorsi:	Lee Haney, Dorian Yates
Gastroc-soleus:	Mike Matarazzo, Vince Taylor

Even though you may not be blessed with the muscle belly lengths of Shawn Ray or Vince Taylor, you can still grow bigger and stronger. The principles in this course will help you reach your limits in the most efficient manner.

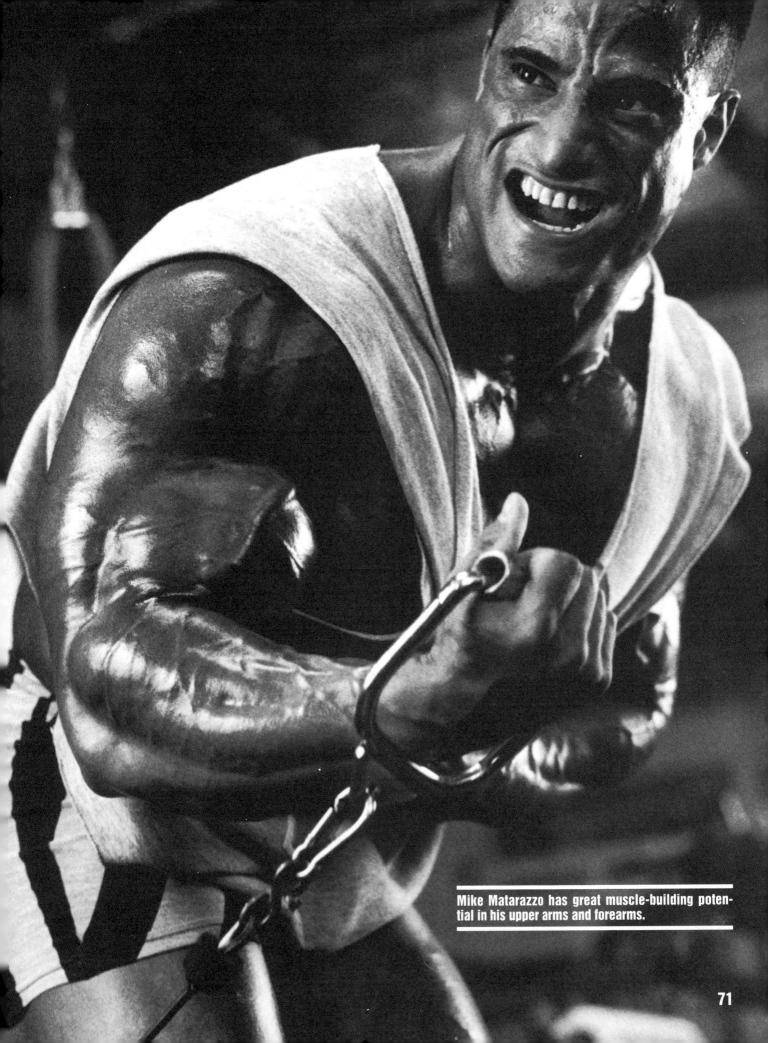

Mike Matarazzo has great muscle-building potential in his upper arms and forearms.

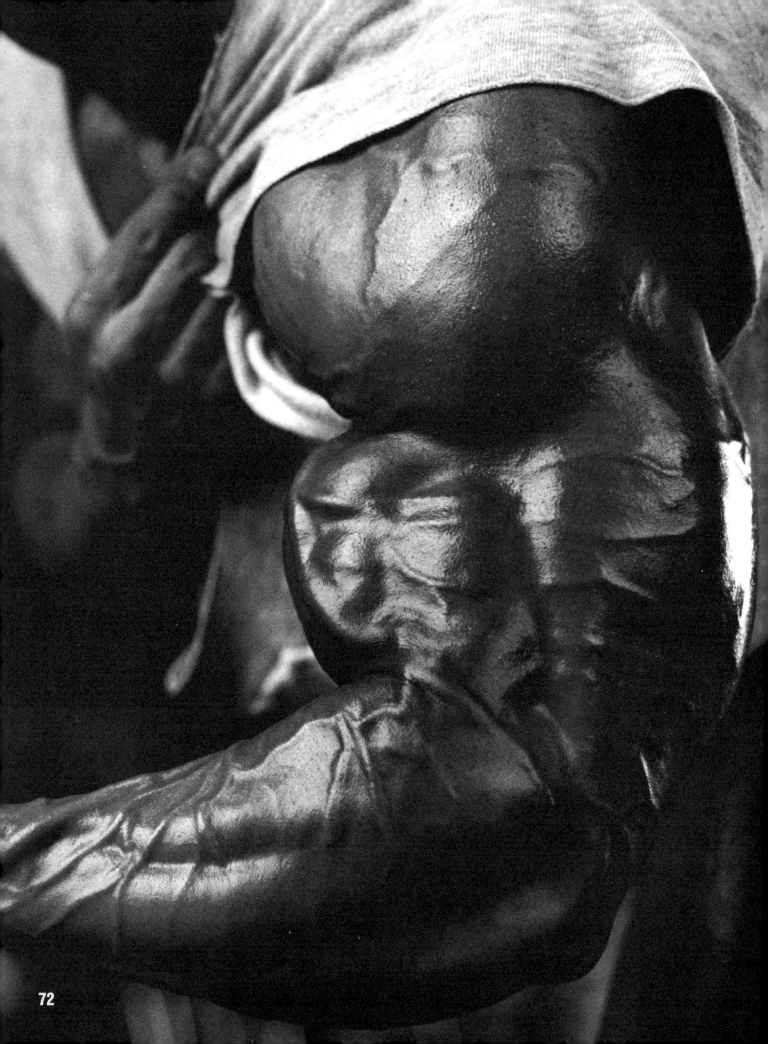

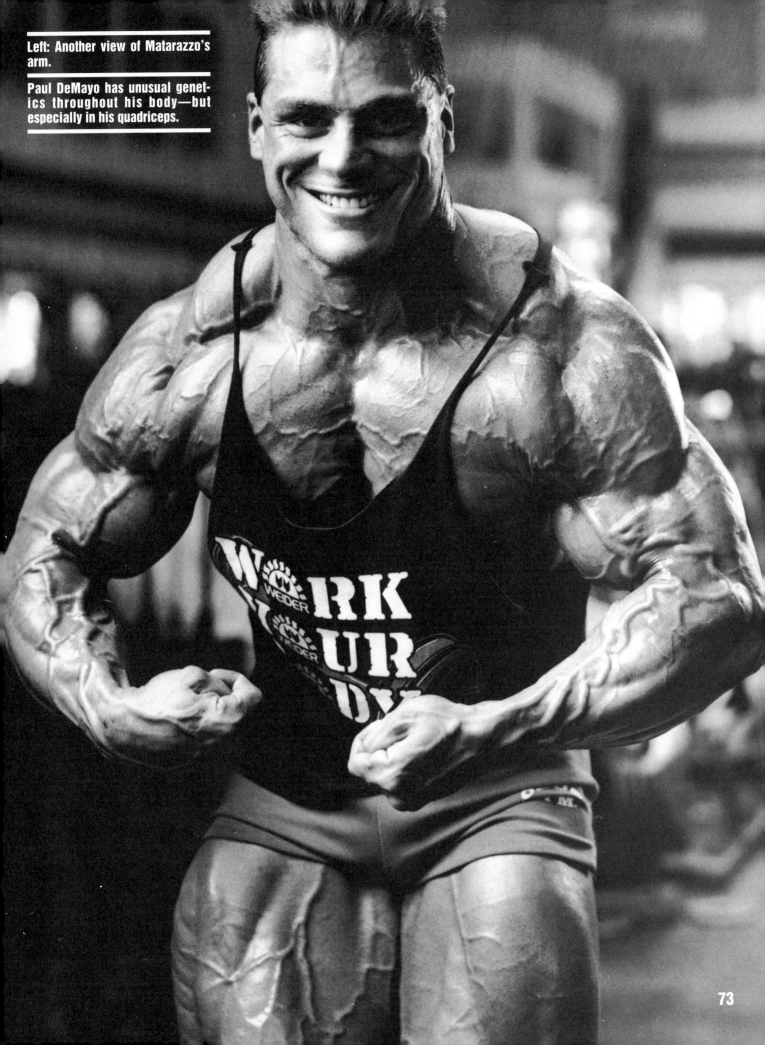

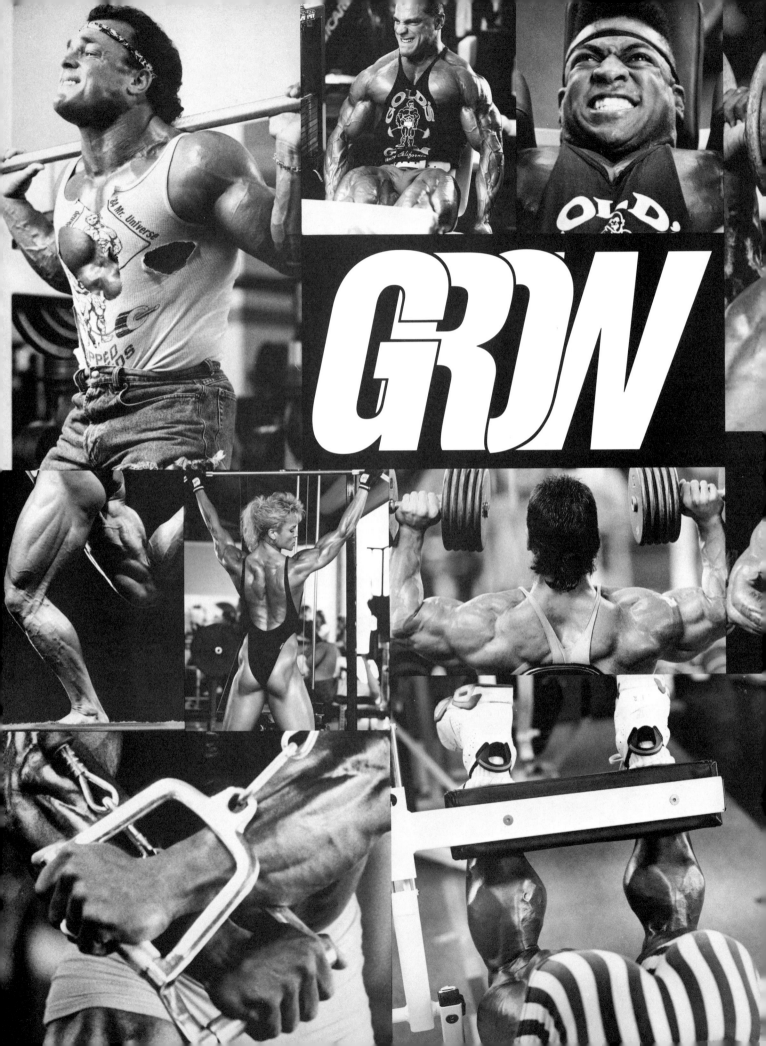

GROW

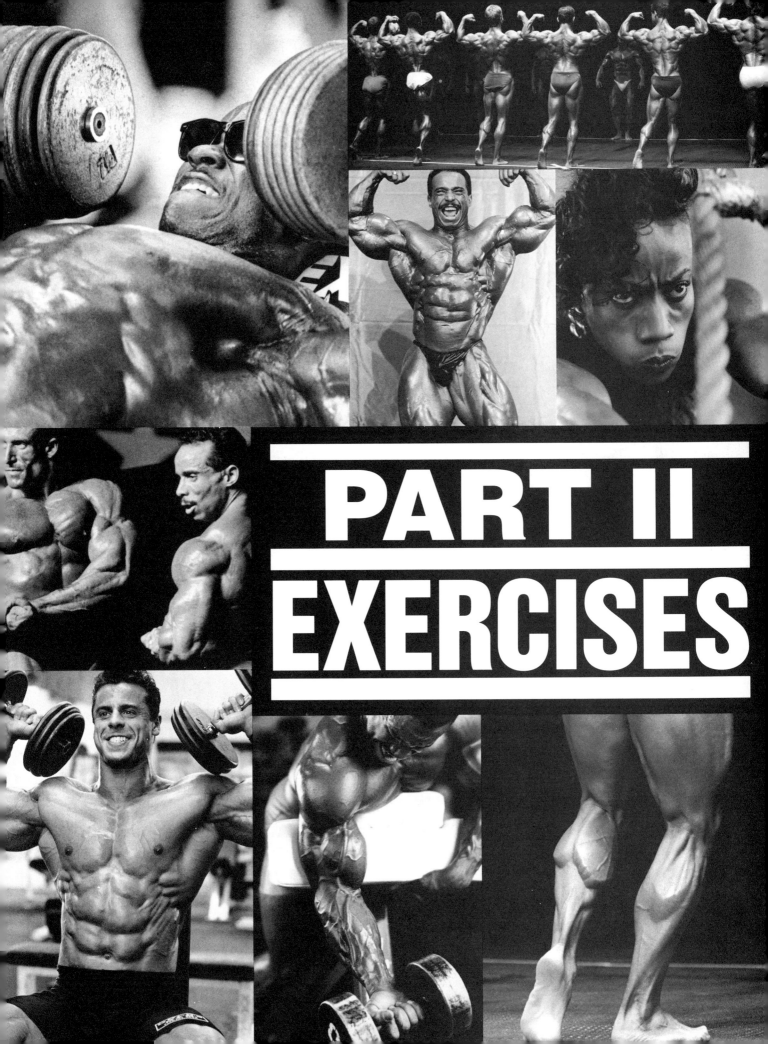

PART II
EXERCISES

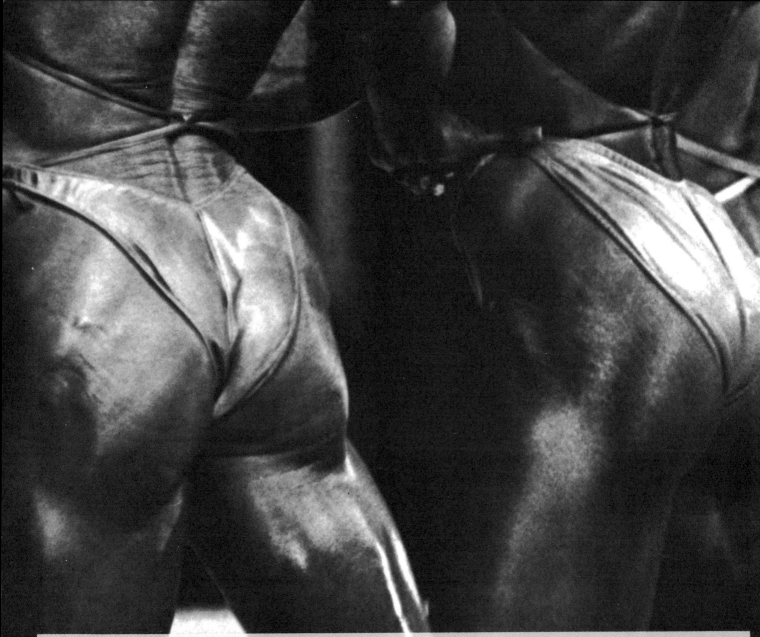

17 • GLUTEALS

The gluteals—composed of the gluteus maximus, gluteus medius, and gluteus minimus—are the largest and thickest muscle group of your body. The major functions of your gluteals are hip extension and hip abduction. Hip extension involves moving the thighs from a flexed, near-your-chest, position to a position beyond your buttocks. Hip abduction refers to spreading the thighs apart laterally.

To develop your gluteals you must do exercises that extend and abduct your hips. The three best exercises for these functions are as follows:

Hip and back machine. Hip extension machines are manufactured by Nautilus, Hammer, and MedX; this description applies to the Nautilus machine. Lie on your back with both legs over the dual roller pads. Fasten the restraining belt across your hips and grasp the handles lightly. Extend both legs smoothly. Keep one leg at full extension. Allow your other knee to bend and your thigh to come back near your chest. Push out with your bent leg until it joins your other leg in the extended position. Pause, arch your lower back, and contract your buttocks. Repeat with other leg. Continue alternating one leg with the other for as many repetitions as possible in proper form.

Hip abduction machine. Sit in the machine and place your legs on the movement arms with your knees together. Push your knees and thighs apart to their widest lateral position. Pause. Return to the knees-together position and repeat.

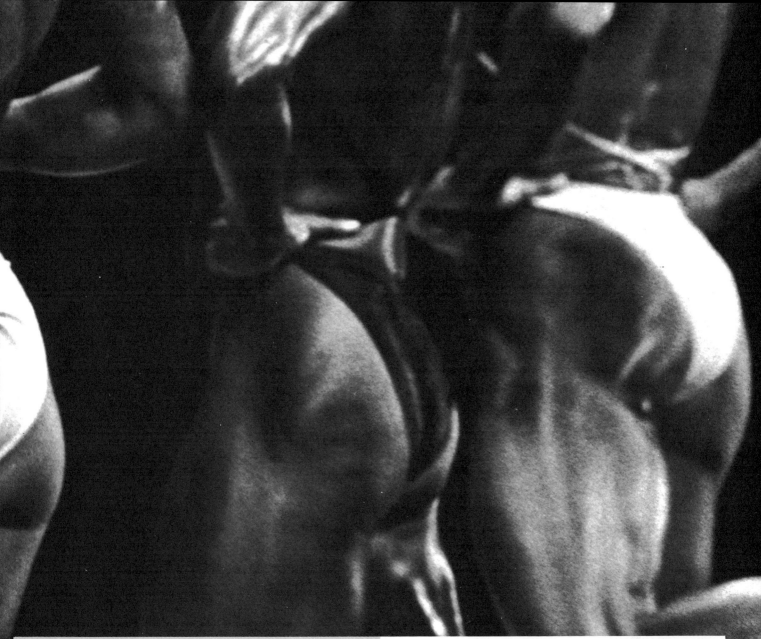

Squat with barbell. The squat not only is a great exercise for your buttocks and thighs but also stimulates growth throughout your body. Place a barbell on a squat rack and load it with an appropriate amount of weight. Position the bar behind your neck across your shoulders and hold the bar in place with your hands. Lift the bar off the rack and step back. Station your feet shoulder-width apart, toes angled slightly outward. Keep your upper body muscles rigid and your torso upright during the exercise. Bend your hips and knees and descend until your hamstrings come in contact with your calves. Without bouncing and without stopping in the bottom position, smoothly return to the top. Repeat.

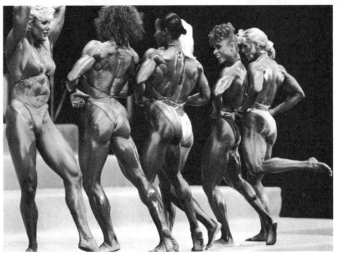

The muscles of the buttocks are the thickest in the body.

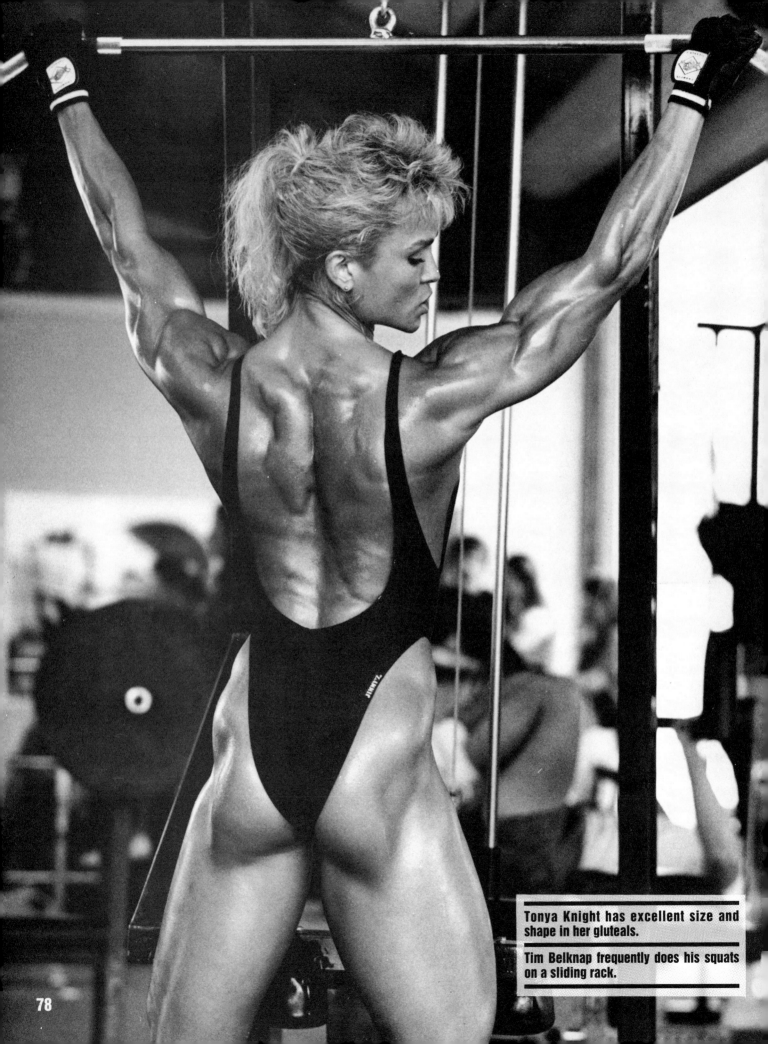

Tonya Knight has excellent size and shape in her gluteals.

Tim Belknap frequently does his squats on a sliding rack.

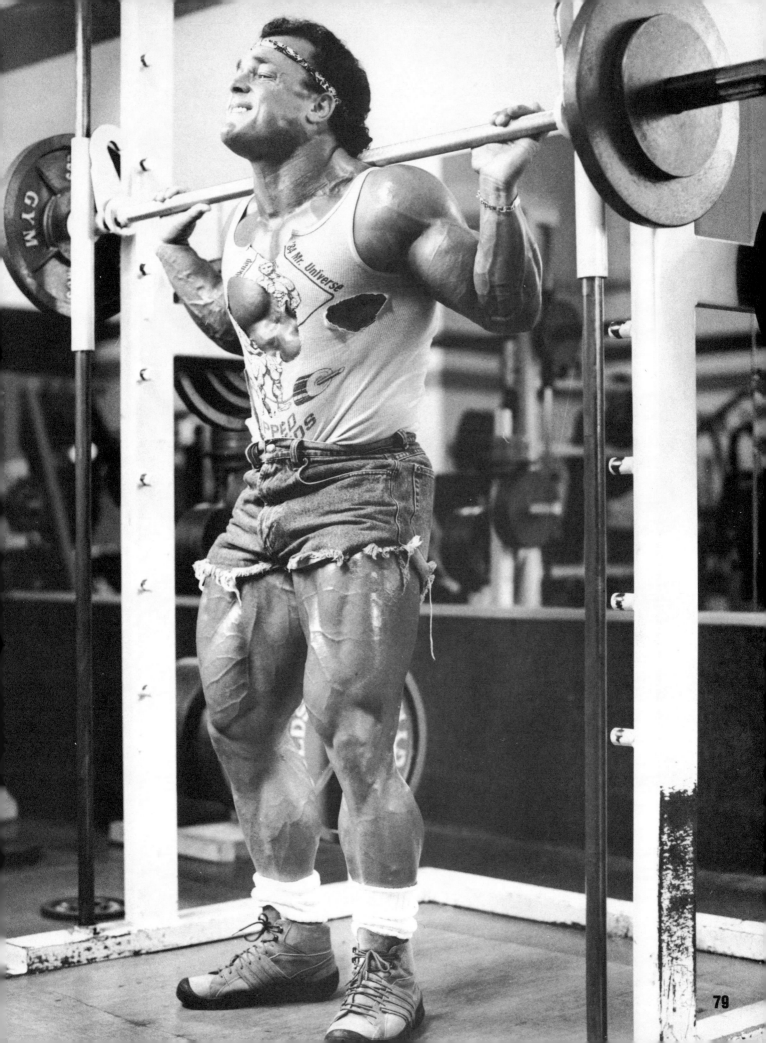

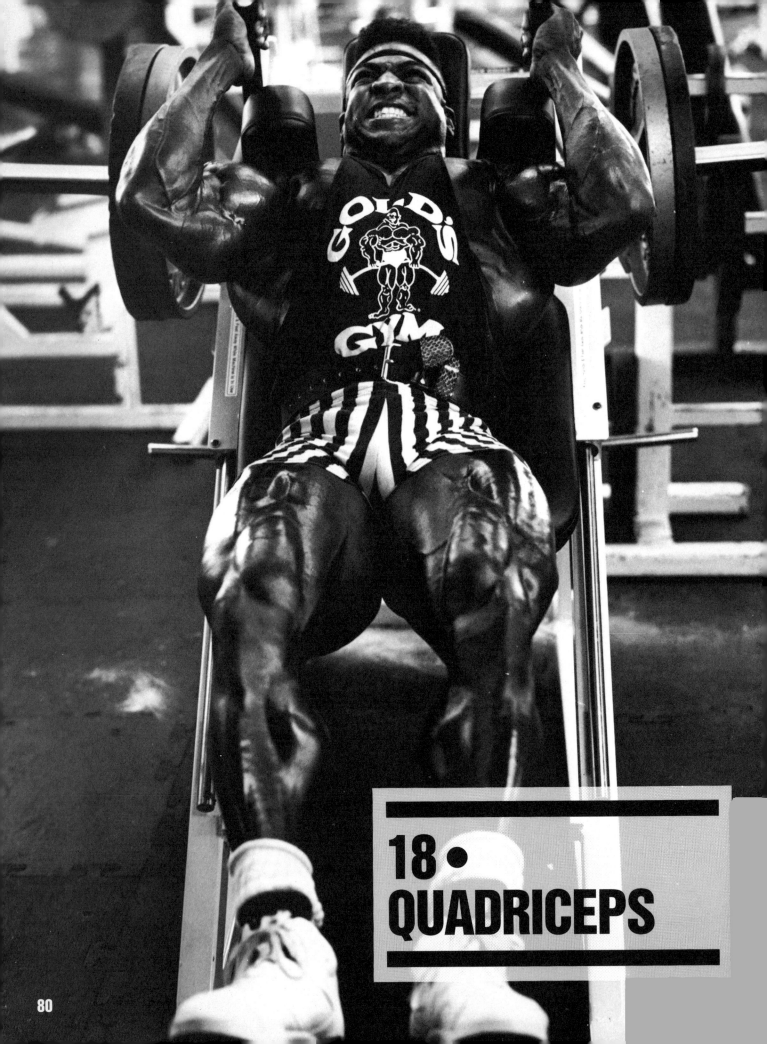

18 • QUADRICEPS

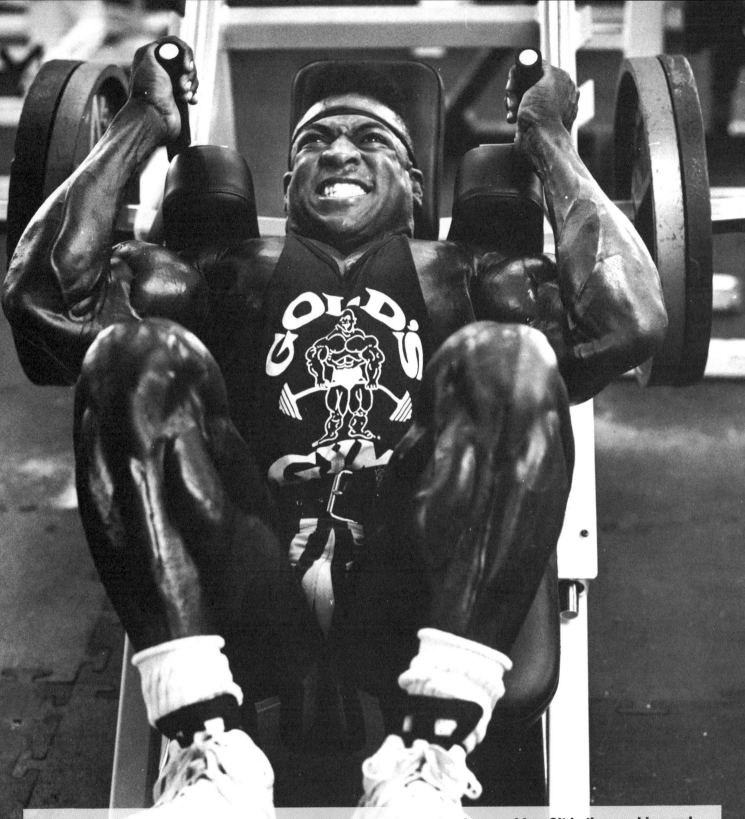

The most important muscles of your front thighs are the quadriceps. The quadriceps are made up of the vastus lateralis, vastus intermedius, vastus medialis, and rectus femoris. The lower tendons of the quadriceps muscles cross your knee joint. Full contraction of your quadriceps causes your knee to extend and your leg to straighten.

The leg extension and the leg press are the recommended exercises for your quadriceps.

Leg extension machine. Sit in the machine and place your ankles behind the bottom roller pads. If possible, align the axis of rotation of the movement arm with your knees. If a belt is provided, strap it tightly across your hips to keep your buttocks from

The angled squat machine takes some of the stress off your lower back.

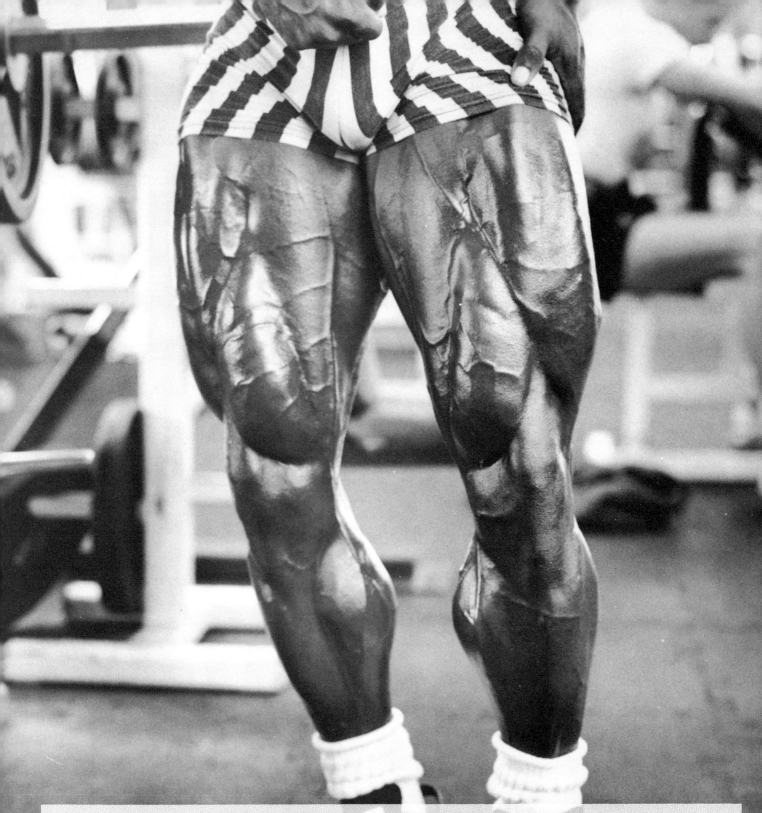

rising. Lean back and stabilize your upper body by grasping the handles. Straighten your legs slowly and ease into the fully contracted top position. Pause briefly. Lower slowly to the bottom. Repeat for maximum repetitions.

Leg press machine. The leg press is a multiple-joint movement that involves the quadriceps, hamstrings, and gluteals. Sit in the machine with your back against the angled pad and your buttocks on the seat bottom. Place your feet on the movable platform with your heels about shoulder-width apart and your toes pointed slightly outward. Straighten your legs smoothly but do not let your knees lock out. Keep a bend of 15 degrees in your knees. Lower smoothly to the bottom position. Do as many repetitions as possible.

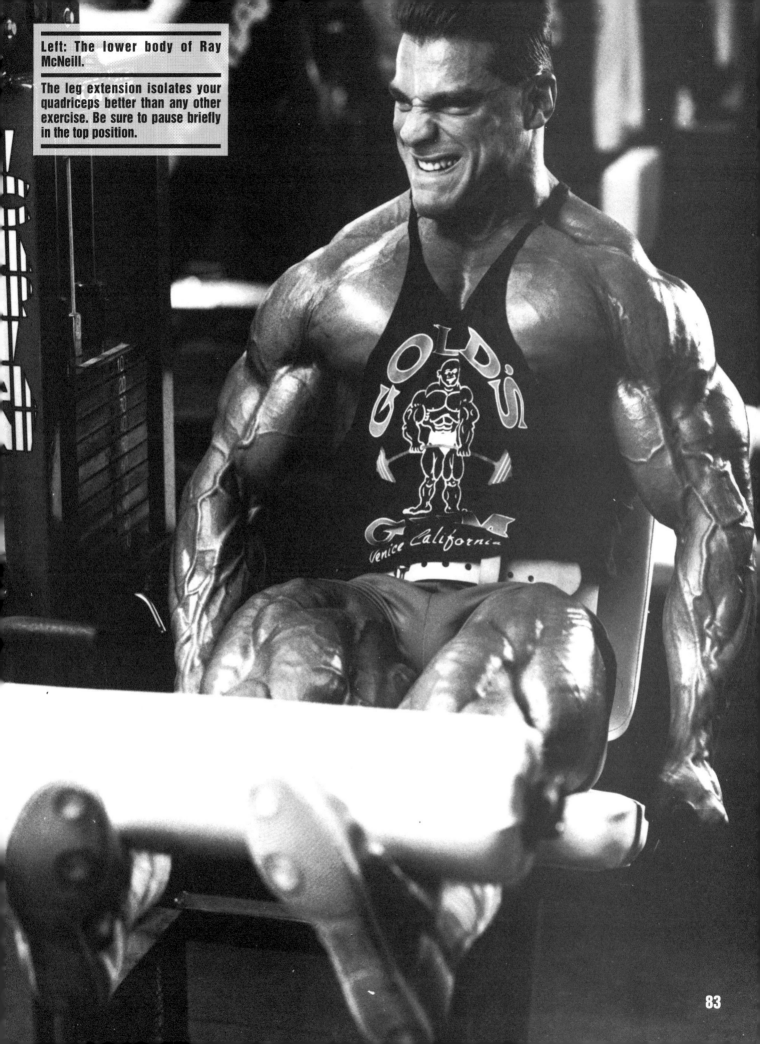

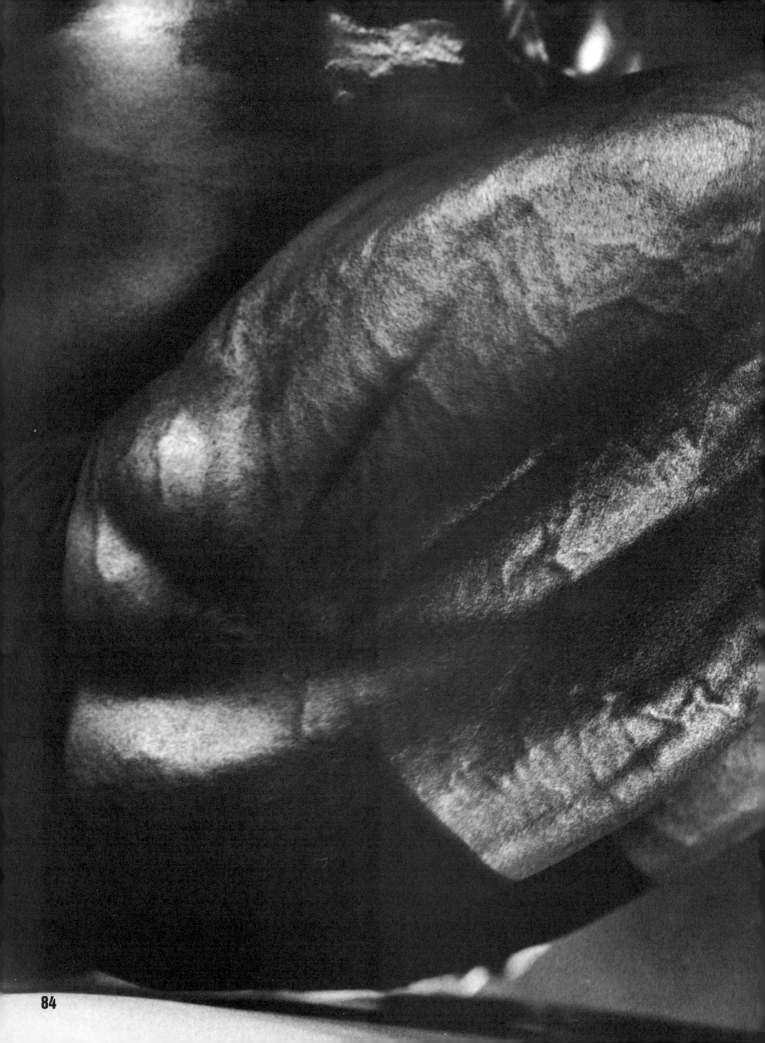

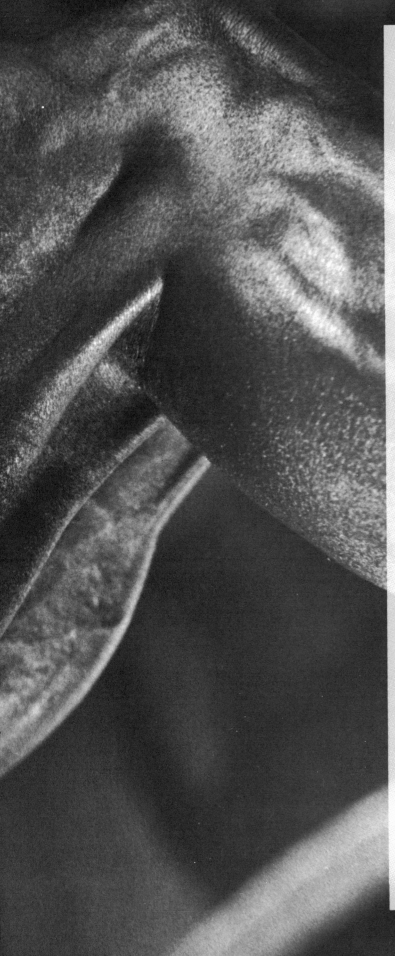

19 •
HAMSTRINGS

Your hamstrings are located in your back thighs. Individual muscles are the semitendinosus, semimembranosus, and biceps femoris. The lower tendons of these three muscles cross the knee joint on the back side. When these muscles contract they bend your knee.

Beside your hamstrings and quadriceps, other important thigh muscles are located on the medial, or inner, section of your thighs. Of these muscles, the adductor magnus is the largest. Your adductor magnus brings your thighs from a spread-legged to a knees-together position. This movement is referred to as hip adduction.

Let's examine the correct use of the leg curl and hip adduction machines.

<u>Leg curl machine.</u> Lie face down on the machine with your knees on the pad edge closest to the movement arm. Hook your heels under the roller pads. Make certain your knees are in line with the axis of rotation of the machine. Grasp the handles provided under the machine bench to steady your upper body. Curl your heels smoothly and try to touch your buttocks. Pause. Lower slowly for a stretch. Repeat until you reach momentary muscular fatigue.

<u>Hip adduction machine.</u> Sit in machine and place your knees and ankles on the movement arms in a spread-legged position. Pull your knees and thighs together smoothly. For better muscle isolation, pull with your thighs—not your ankles and lower legs. Pause in the knees-together position. Return slowly for a stretch. Repeat.

The leg press not only involves the quadriceps but also the hamstrings.

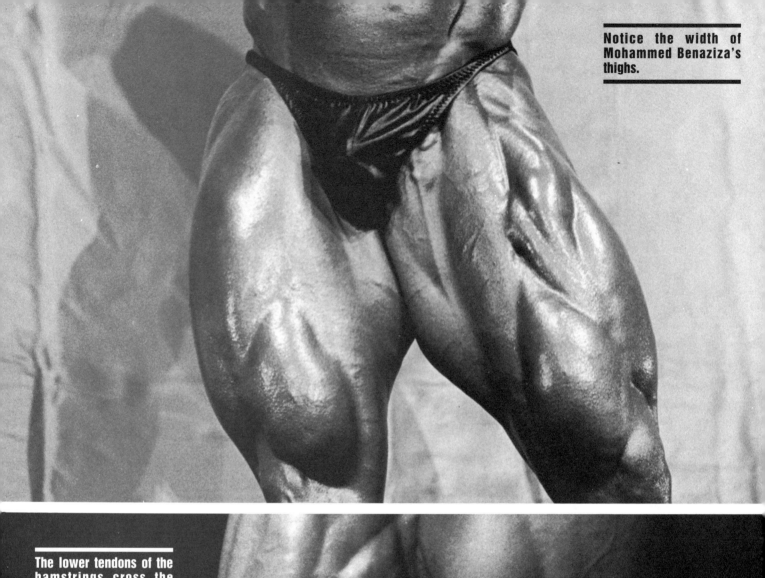

Notice the width of Mohammed Benaziza's thighs.

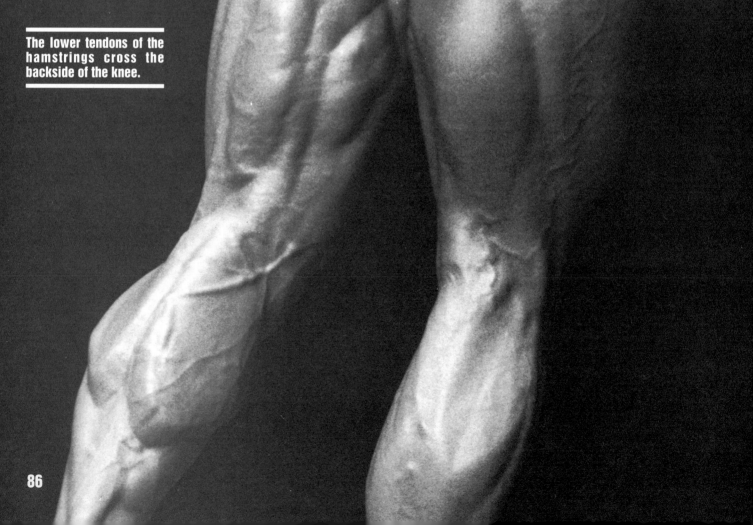

The lower tendons of the hamstrings cross the backside of the knee.

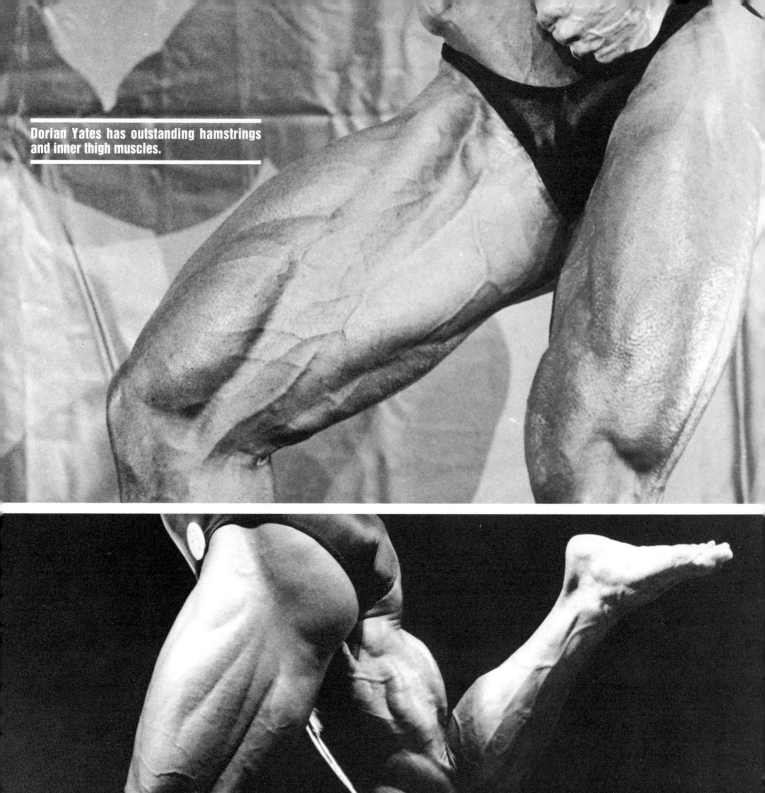

Dorian Yates has outstanding hamstrings and inner thigh muscles.

Knee flexion is the primary function of the hamstrings.

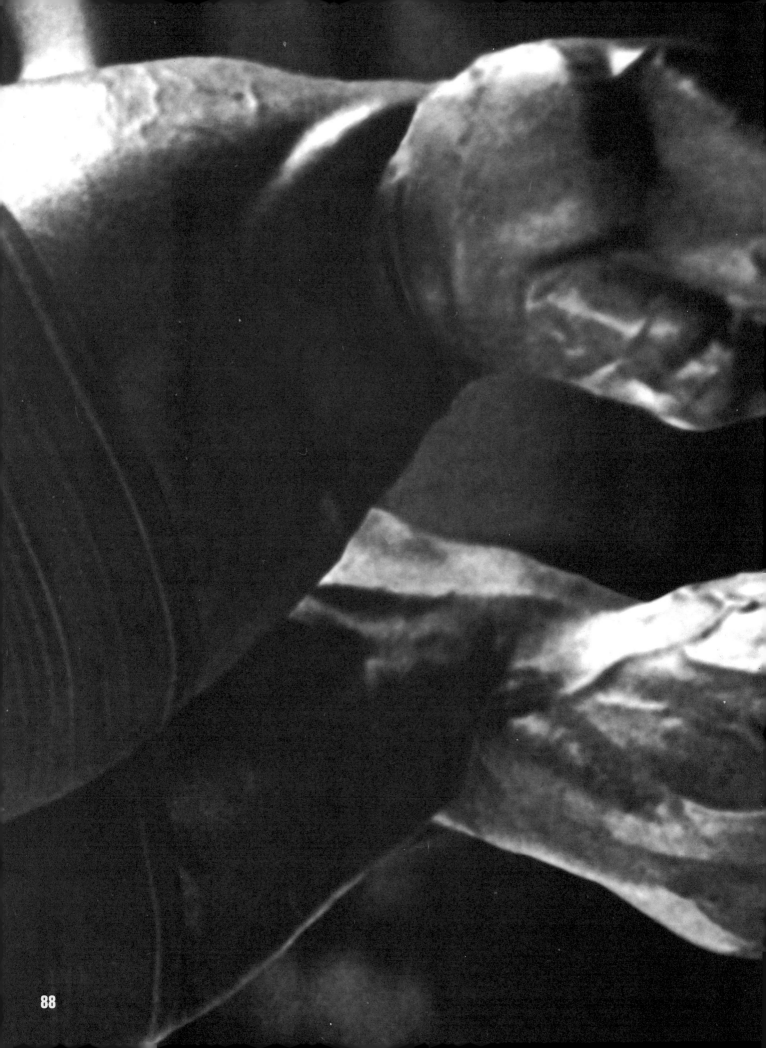

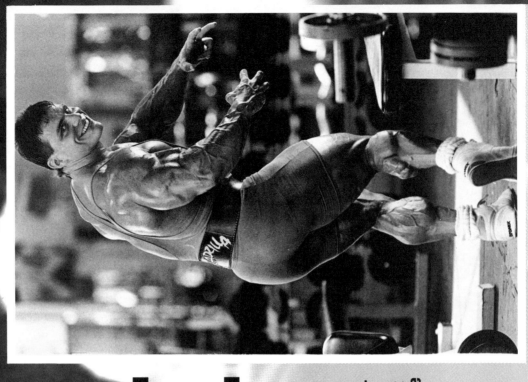

Your calves can be the focal point of your body from the back-side. Don't neglect them.

20 • GASTROC-SOLEUS

The most important muscles of your back calf are the gastrocnemius and soleus. The gastrocnemius is the large U-shaped muscle at the back of your lower leg. Underneath the gastrocnemius is a long flat muscle called the soleus.

When these muscles contract, your foot extends. If you are standing, your heel is lifted from the floor. Your soleus, however, does most of the extending when your knee is flexed to 90 degrees or more.

For complete lower leg development, you must do both standing and seated calf raises. Here are the specifics on each exercise:

Standing calf raise machine. Stand under the calf machine with the balls of your feet securely on a block or step. Straighten your knees and keep them locked throughout the exercise. Sag your heels as far below the level of your toes as comfortably possible. Keep your feet pointed straight ahead. Raise your heels smoothly and try to stand on your tiptoes. Pause briefly in the highest position. Lower slowly and repeat.

Seated calf raise machine. Sit in the machine and adjust the padded movement arm so your knees fit snugly underneath. Only the balls of your feet should be on the lower step. Raise your heels and stand on your tiptoes. Pause. Lower slowly and stretch. Repeat for maximum repetitions.

89

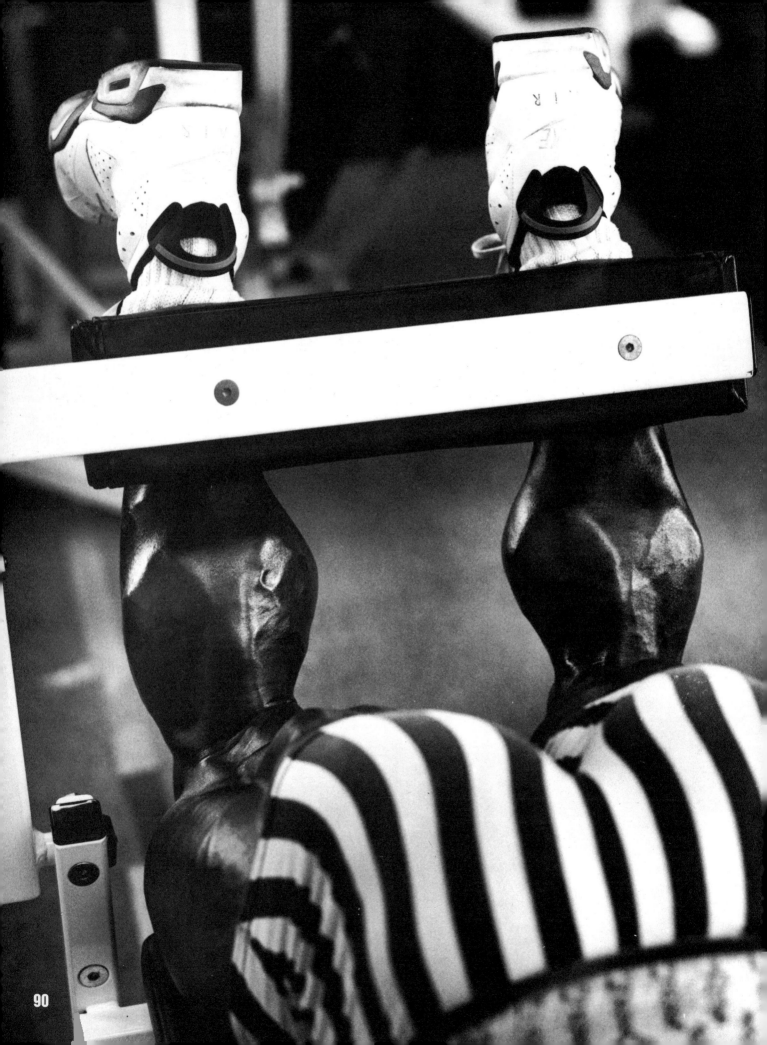

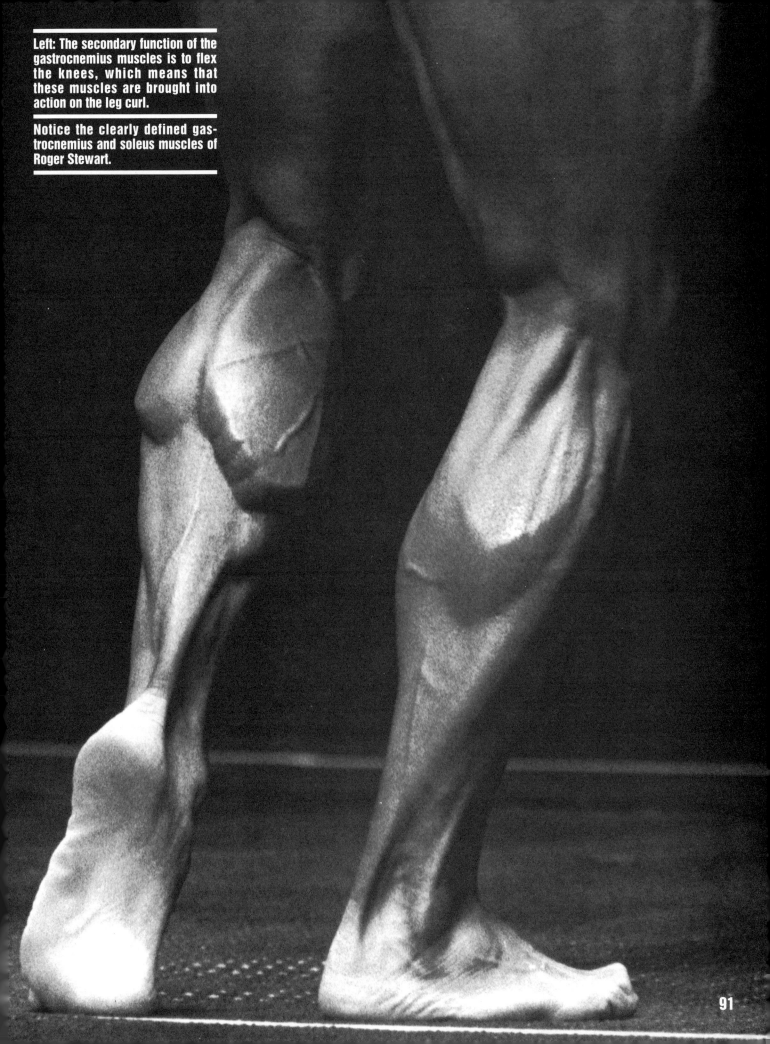

Left: The secondary function of the gastrocnemius muscles is to flex the knees, which means that these muscles are brought into action on the leg curl.

Notice the clearly defined gastrocnemius and soleus muscles of Roger Stewart.

21 • DELTOIDS

You can never get your shoulders too broad. But if you could, then the mass of your deltoids would be to blame.

The deltoid, a triangular muscle, is on the shoulder with one angle pointing down the arm and the other two bent around your shoulder to the front and rear. When the deltoid contracts, it lifts your upper arm forward, sideways, or backward.

The best exercises for your deltoids are dumbbell raises and overhead presses.

Lateral raise with dumbbells. Grasp a dumbbell in each hand and stand. Lock your elbows and wrists and keep them locked throughout the exercise. Raise your arms sideways smoothly. Pause briefly when the dumbbells are slightly higher than horizontal. Make sure your palms are facing down and your elbows are straight. Lower slowly to your sides and repeat.

Overhead press with barbell. In a standing position with your hands shoulder-width apart on a barbell, press the barbell in front of your face and over your head. Do not lock your elbows—keep them slightly bent at the top. Lower the barbell smoothly to your shoulders. Repeat until you reach momentary fatigue.

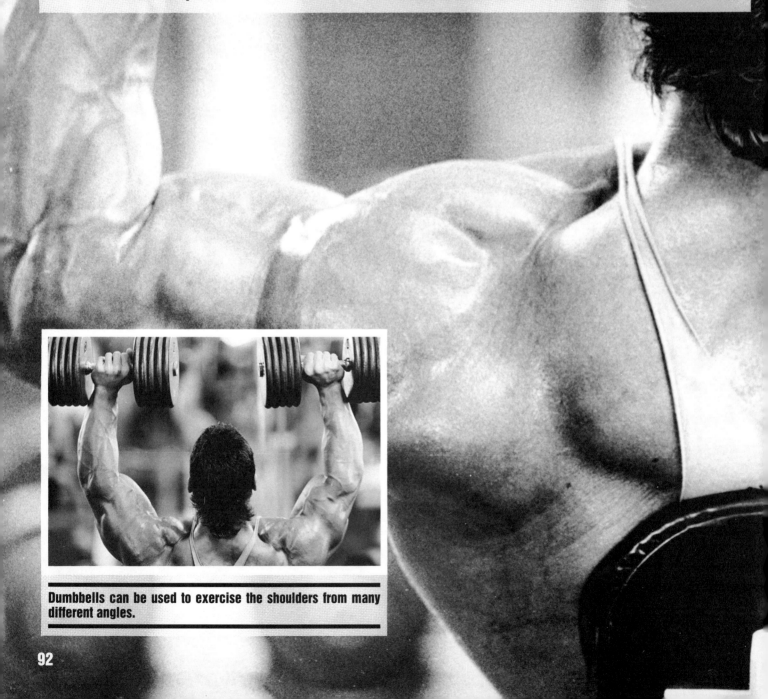

Dumbbells can be used to exercise the shoulders from many different angles.

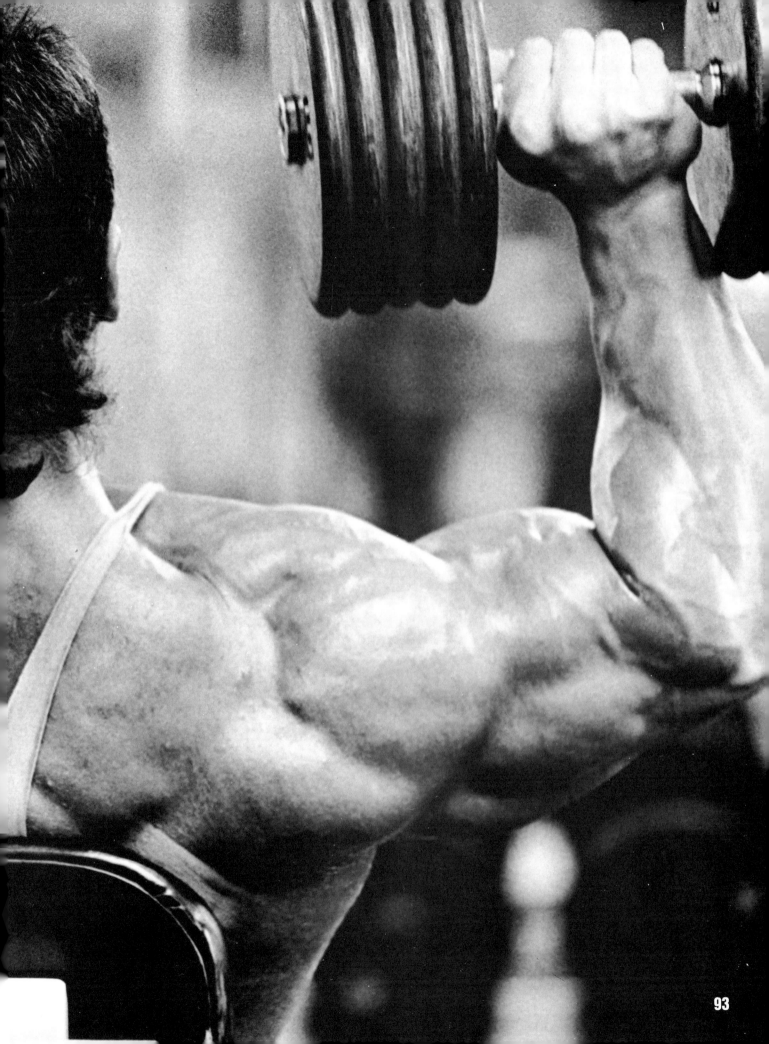

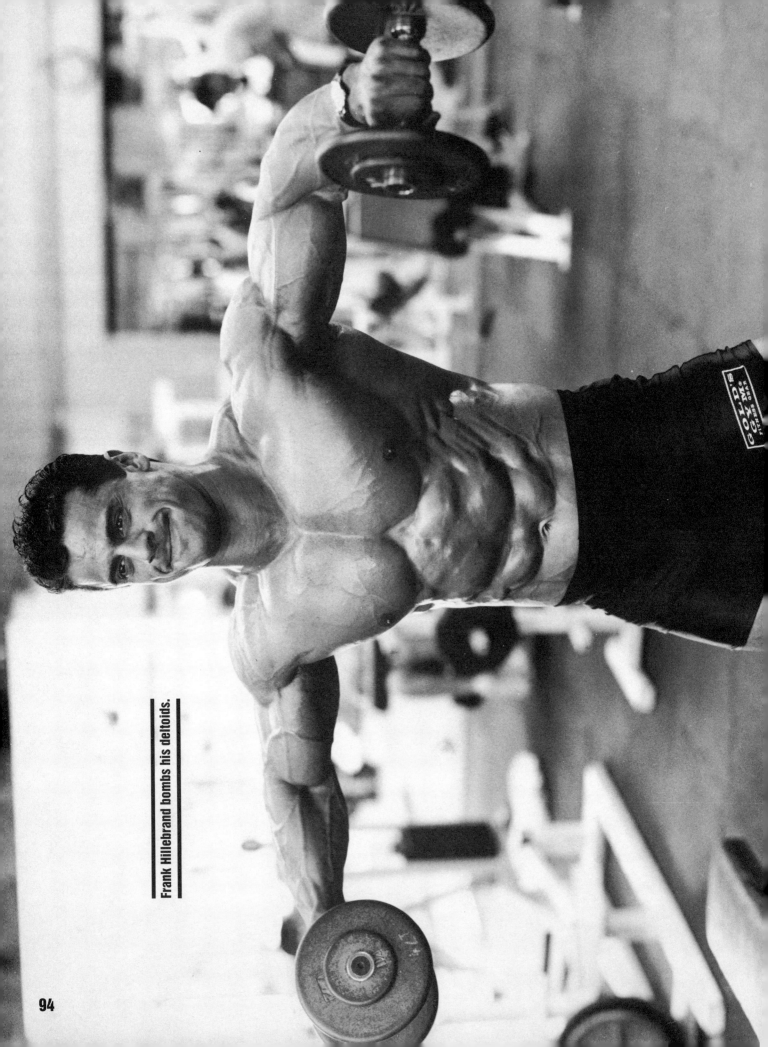

Frank Hillebrand bombs his deltoids.

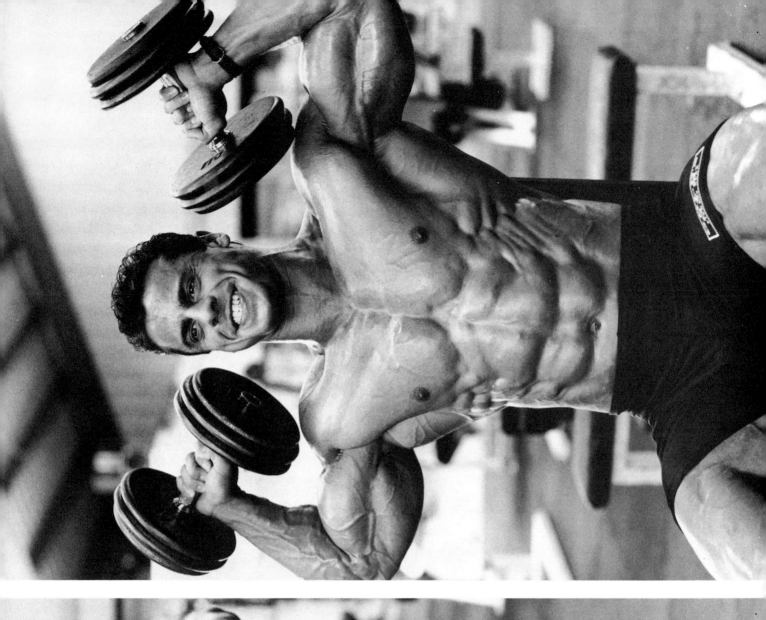

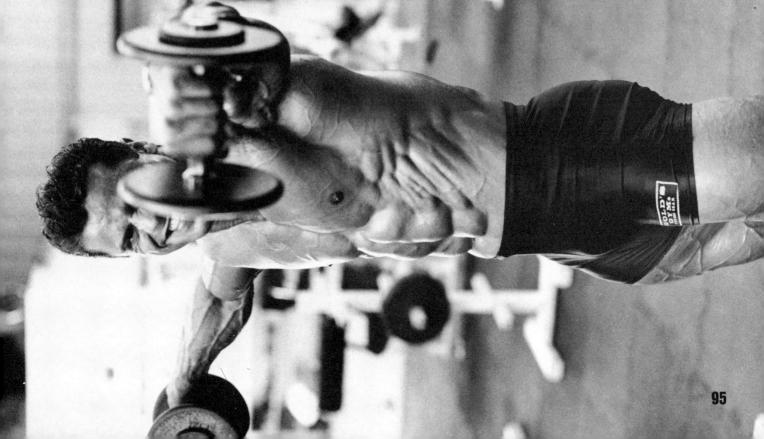

22 •
LATISSIMUS DORSI

Well-developed latissimus dorsi muscles give your upper body the much-admired V shape. The latissimus dorsi are situated primarily on the lower two-thirds of your back. These very wide muscles insert on your upper arms. Thus, when they contract they pull your upper arms from an overhead position down and around your shoulder axes.

The best exercises for the latissimus dorsi, then, must involve pullover, rowing, and pulldown actions. Here are the recommended movements:

Pullover on machine. Nautilus still manufactures the best pullover machine. The resistance is placed directly on the upper arms, as it should be for muscle isolation. Adjust the seat until your shoulders are aligned with the axes of rotation of the movement arm. Fasten the seat belt tightly across your hips. Depress the foot pedal, place your elbows on the pads, and release the foot pedal. Rotate your elbows back into the stretched position. Pull your elbows forward and down until the movement arm touches your midsection. Pause. Return slowly to the stretched position. Repeat for maximum repetitions.

Negative pullover on machine. Increase the resistance approximately 40 percent above what you would normally handle. You'll need one or two helpers to assist you in moving the bar into the fully contracted position during the positive portion of the pullover. It is important that your assistants make the transfer smoothly to your arms. Pause in the fully contracted position and slowly rotate your arms to the stretched position. The slow negative rotation should take 10 seconds. On your cue, the assistants should grasp the movement arm and bring it down to the contracted

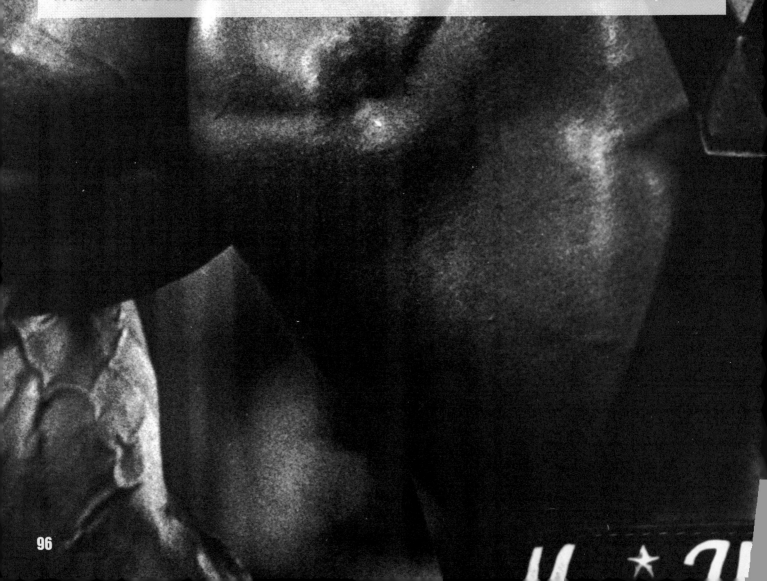

position. Repeat the slow negatives for 8 to 12 repetitions.

Bent-armed pullover with barbell. Lie face up on a high, narrow bench with your head barely off the edge. Anchor your feet securely underneath. Have your training partner hand you a heavy barbell. Your hands should be spaced 12 inches apart. The barbell should be resting on your chest. Move the barbell over your face and head and try to touch the floor. Stretch in the bottom position and smoothly pull the barbell above your face to your chest. Repeat for as many repetitions as possible.

Bent-over row with barbell. In a bent-over position place your hands about four inches apart and use an overhanded grip. Pull the barbell up your thighs smoothly until it touches your waist. Lower smoothly for a stretch. Repeat.

Pulldown on lat machine. Stabilize yourself under the lat machine bar. Grasp the overhead bar with a narrow underhanded grip. Pull the bar smoothly to your chest. Return slowly to the stretched position. Repeat for maximum repetitions.

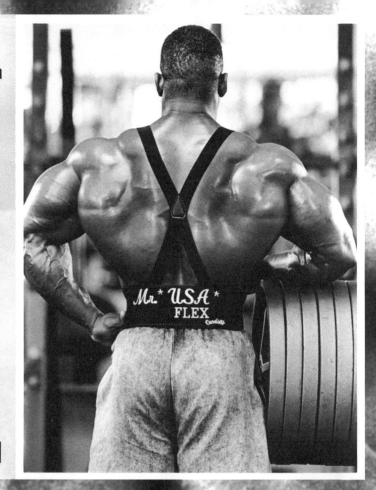

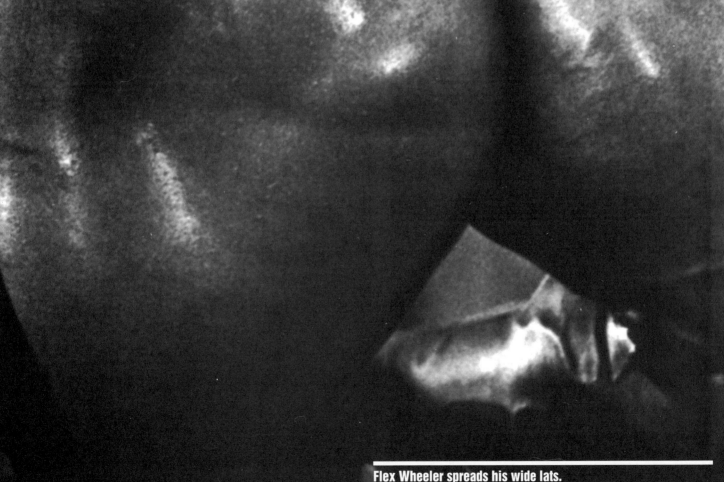

Flex Wheeler spreads his wide lats.

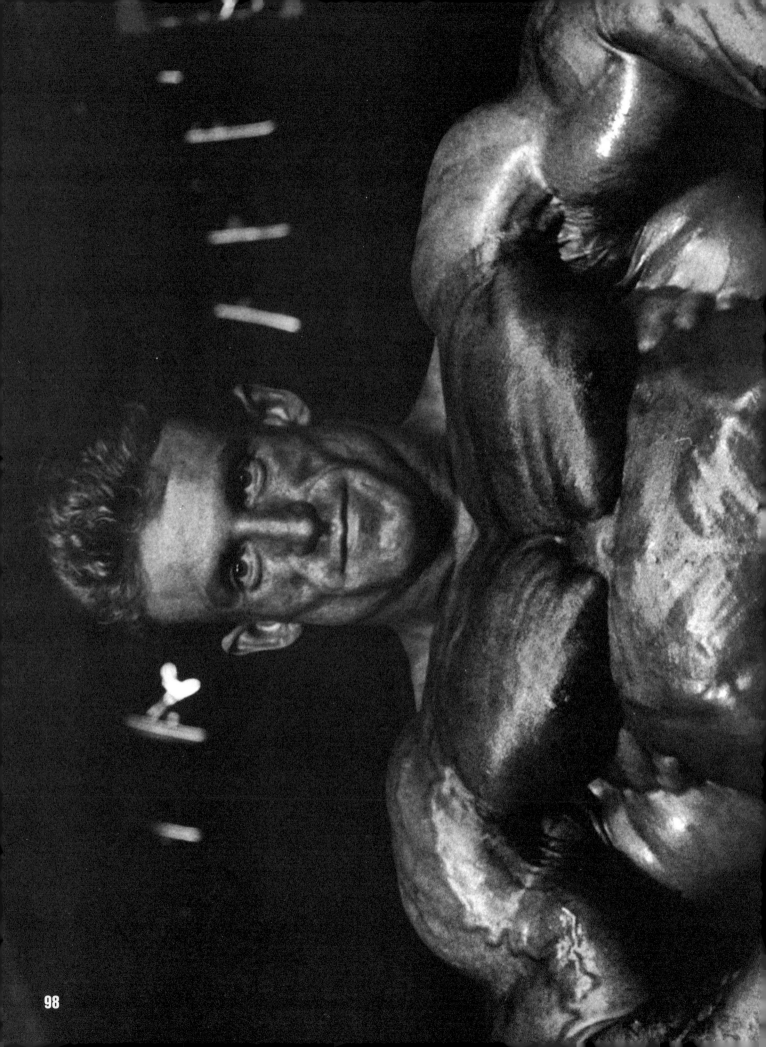

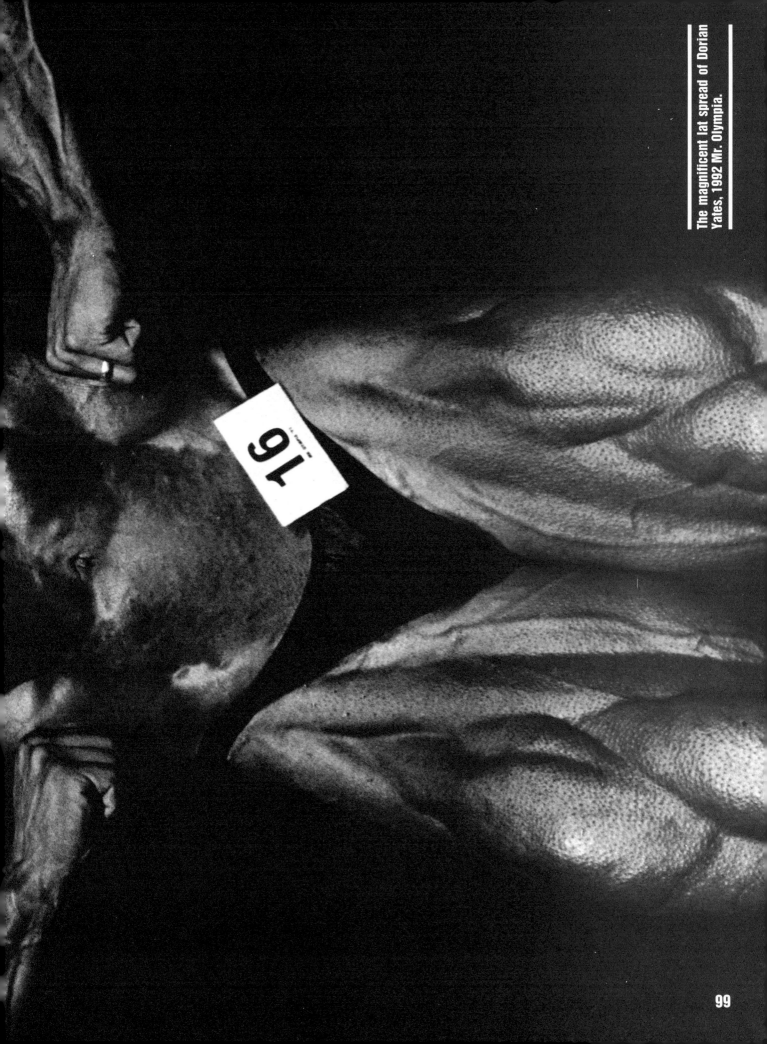

The magnificent lat spread of Dorian Yates, 1992 Mr. Olympia.

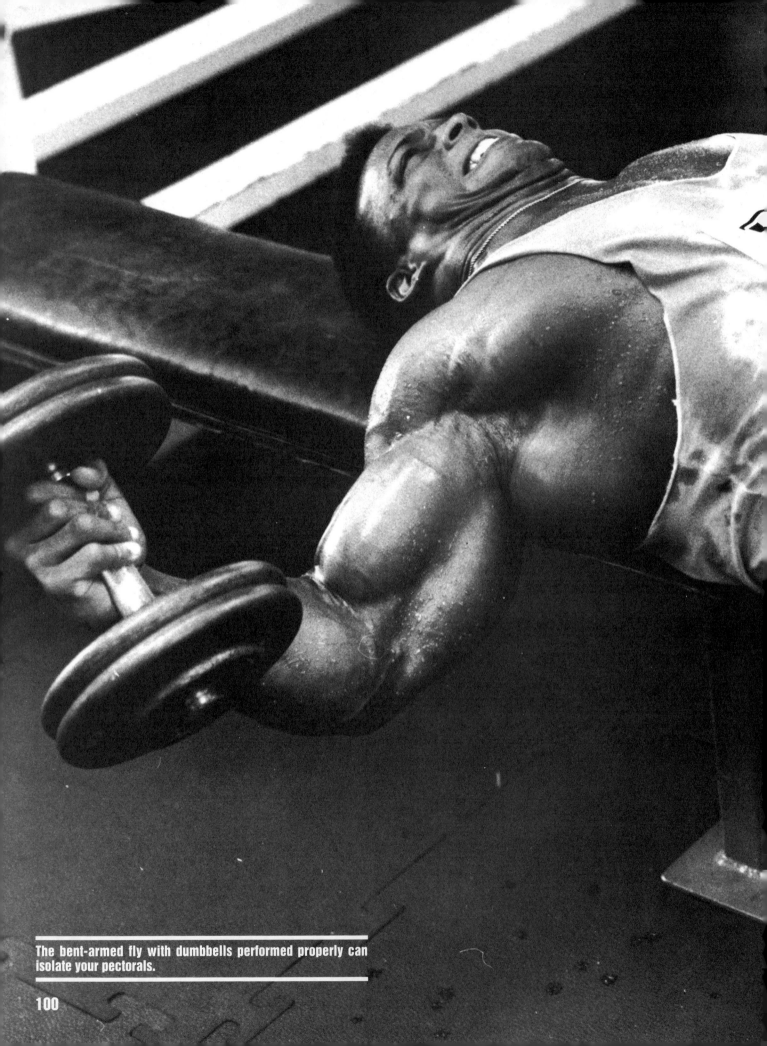

The bent-armed fly with dumbbells performed properly can isolate your pectorals.

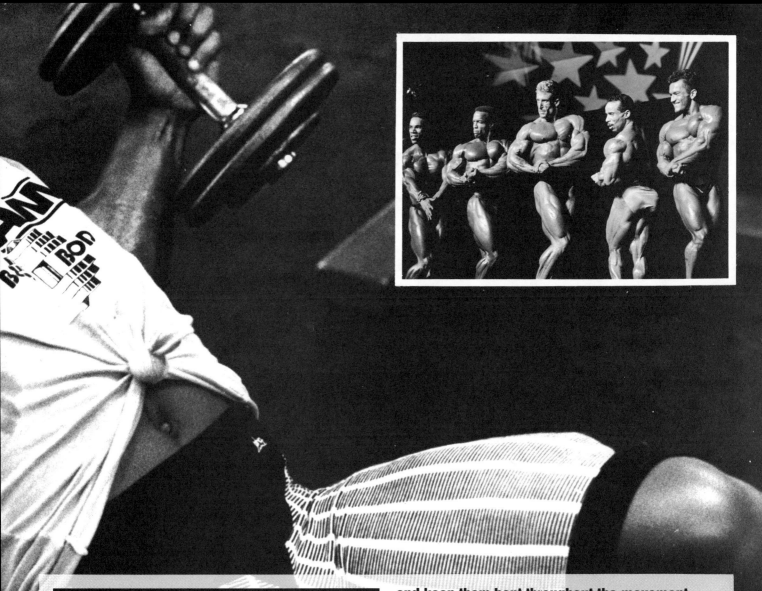

23 • PECTORALS

The pectoralis major is a large fan-shaped muscle lying across the front of your chest. One part of this muscle is attached along the entire length of your sternum and at least half of your clavicle. The other part of the pectoral inserts on the front of your upper-arm bone. When your pectorals contract, they pull your upper arms across your torso.

The recommended exercises for your pectorals are the bent-armed fly, bench press, and incline press. Here's how to perform each one:

Bent-armed fly with dumbbells. Grasp two dumbbells, lie back on a flat exercise bench, and extend your arms upward from your shoulders. Your palms should be facing each other while holding the dumbbells. Bend your elbows slightly and keep them bent throughout the movement. Lower the dumbbells out to your sides in semicircular arcs as low as comfortably possible. Return the dumbbells smoothly along the same arcs to the top position. Repeat for maximum repetitions.

Bench press with barbell. For safety purposes, it is necessary to have a bench with an attached barbell rack. In a supine position, grasp the barbell with a shoulder-width grip, lift the bar from the rack, and stabilize it over your chest. Lower the barbell slowly to your chest and press it back until your elbows are almost straight. Do as many repetitions as possible.

Incline press with barbell. It's best to have an incline bench with an attached rack for this exercise. Position yourself properly on the bench and lift the barbell off the rack to a stable position. Lower the barbell slowly to your upper chest. Press it smoothly back until your elbows are almost straight. Repeat.

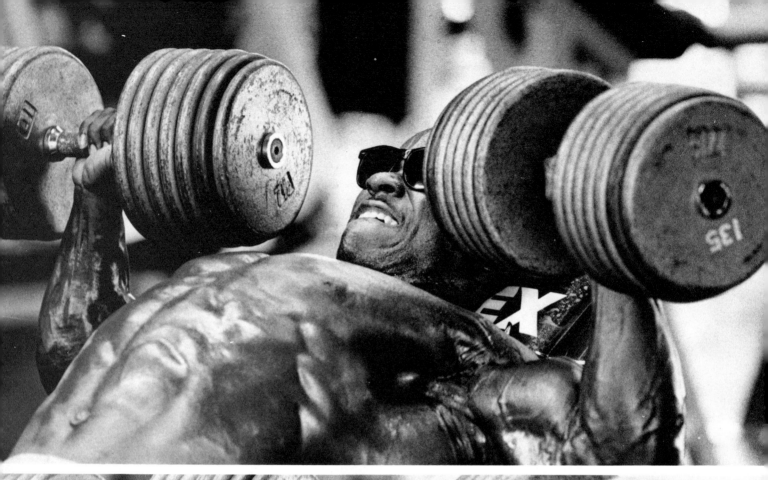

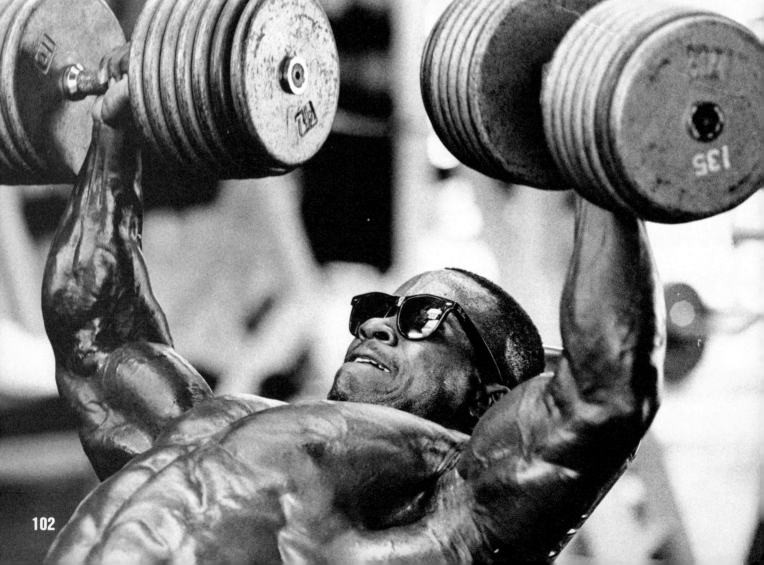

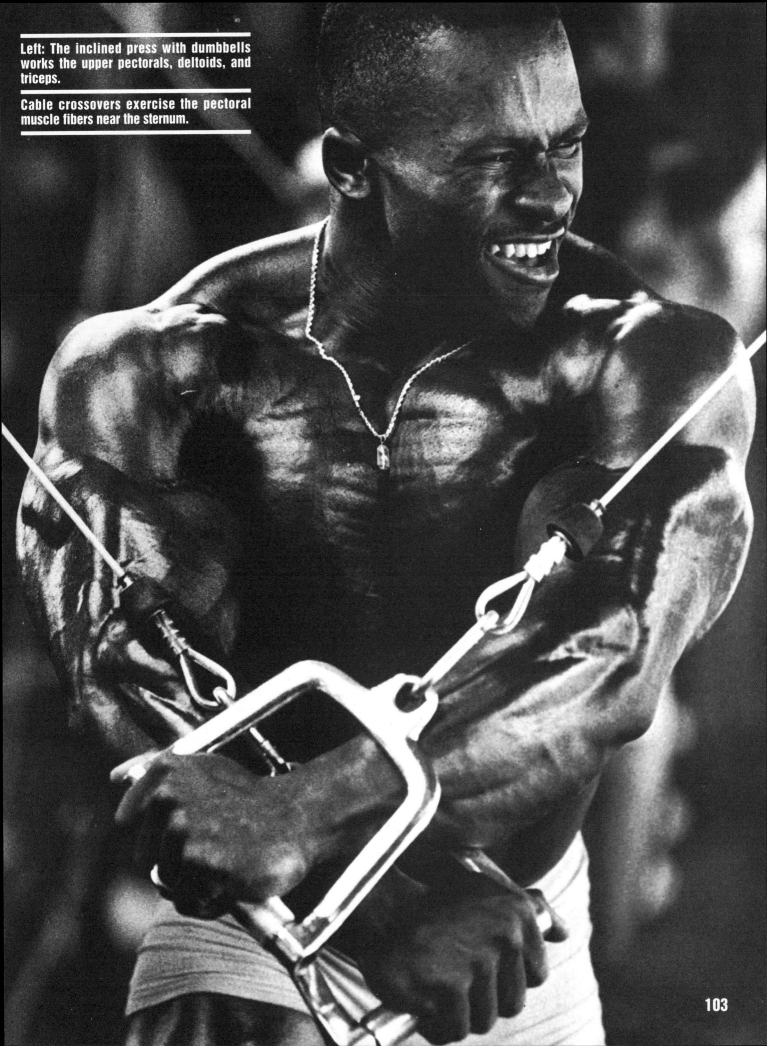

Left: The inclined press with dumbbells works the upper pectorals, deltoids, and triceps.

Cable crossovers exercise the pectoral muscle fibers near the sternum.

24 • ERECTOR SPINAE

The erector spinae are a series of long, deep muscles that extend from your sacrum to your skull on both sides of your spine. When these muscles contract they extend your spine backward.

Few bodybuilders have thick, well-developed erector spinae muscles. It's a shame, because these muscles add extra dimensions to the body's backside.

Suggested exercises for your erector spinae muscles are the stiff-legged deadlift, the 4-way neck machine, and the shoulder shrug. While the shoulder shrug does not directly extend the spine, it adds stability and strength to your shoulder girdle and neck.

Stiff-legged deadlift. Be sure to do this exercise with a slight bend in your knees—this protects the vertebrae of your lower back. Stand with your feet under a barbell. Bend your knees, grasp the bar with one hand under and the other hand over, and stand up smoothly. Lower the barbell slowly down your thighs while keeping a slight bend in your knees. Stretch in the bottom position. Lift the weight slowly back to an almost-erect position. Do the required repetitions.

4-way neck machine. Nautilus and Hammer make popular versions of this machine, and they are both used in the same way. Your seat position is important in each of the four directions of the exercise: back, front, right, and left. Once the seat level is established for any of the four directions, the same position applies to the other three. When you are seated upright, the pivot point of the movement arm should be aligned with the middle of your throat or Adam's apple. To exercise the back of your neck, sit away from the machine and place the back of your head firmly against the pads. Extend your head as far back as possible. Pause. Lower your head slowly to the stretched position. Repeat. To work the front part of your neck, turn and face the movement

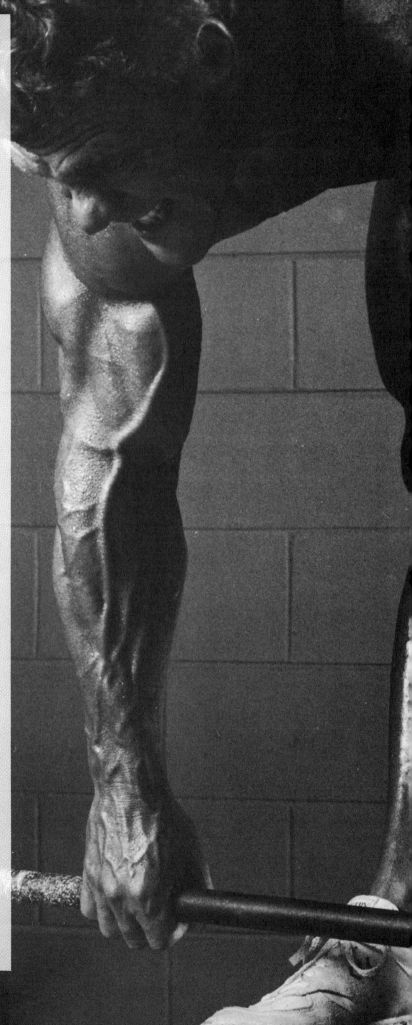

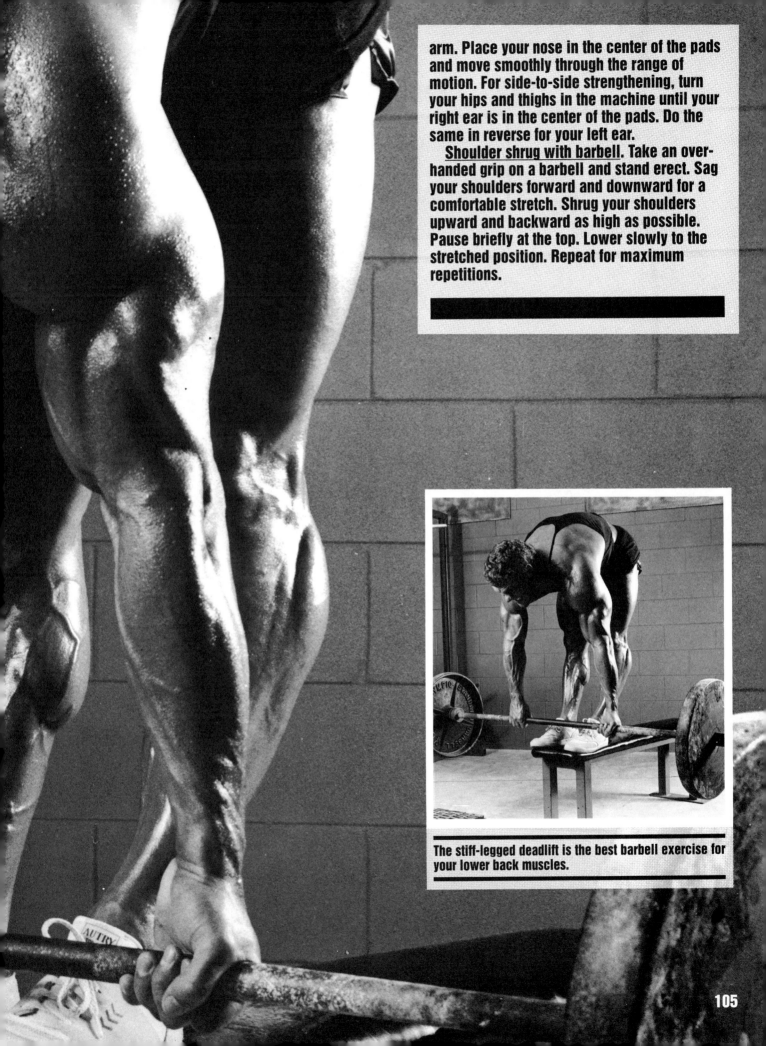

arm. Place your nose in the center of the pads and move smoothly through the range of motion. For side-to-side strengthening, turn your hips and thighs in the machine until your right ear is in the center of the pads. Do the same in reverse for your left ear.

<u>Shoulder shrug with barbell</u>. Take an over-handed grip on a barbell and stand erect. Sag your shoulders forward and downward for a comfortable stretch. Shrug your shoulders upward and backward as high as possible. Pause briefly at the top. Lower slowly to the stretched position. Repeat for maximum repetitions.

The stiff-legged deadlift is the best barbell exercise for your lower back muscles.

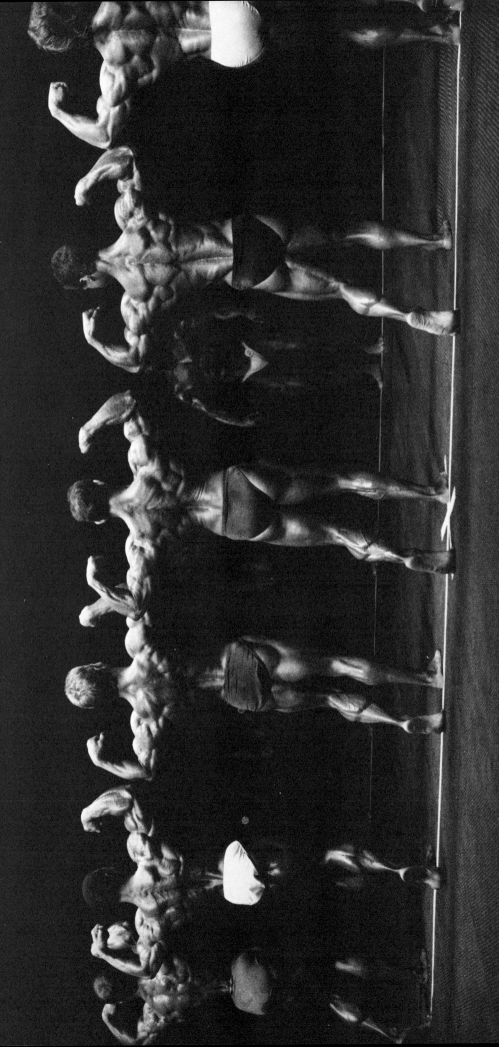

Notice the variation in the back muscles of these contestants.

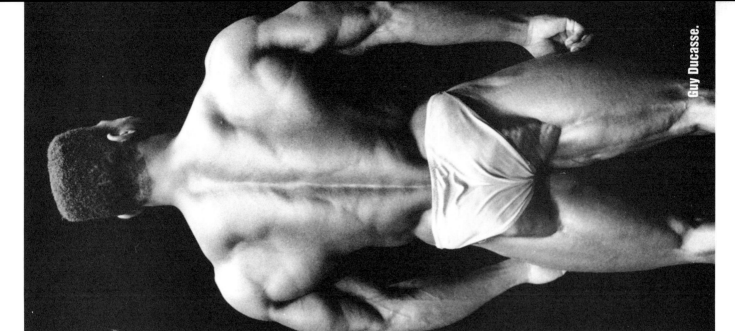

Guy Ducasse.

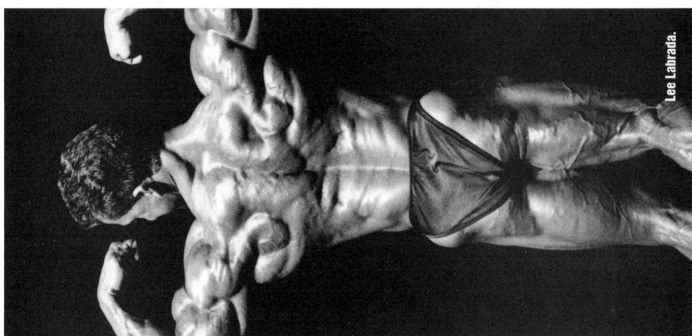

Lee Labrada.

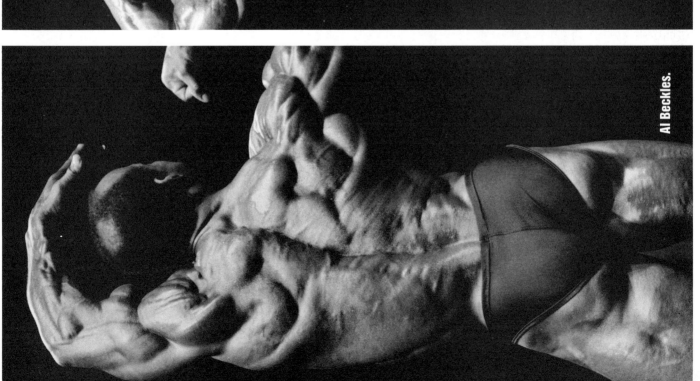

Al Beckles.

25 • BICEPS

All bodybuilders know that the biceps is the most prominent muscle on the front side of the upper arm. What many of these bodybuilders may not know, however, is that the biceps crosses not only the elbow but also the shoulder. As a result, the biceps flexes your elbow and lifts your upper arm forward. But that's not all your biceps does. It supinates your hand. That's why you can curl more resistance with a supinated, palms-up grip than you can with a pronated, palms-down grip.

Here are the best exercises for your biceps as well as a couple of related exercises for your forearms.

Biceps curl with barbell. Take a shoulder-width underhanded grip on a barbell and stand. Anchor your elbows firmly against the sides of your waist and keep them there throughout the exercise. Lean forward slightly with your shoulders. Look down at your hands and curl the bar smoothly. Pause in the top position but do not move your elbows forward. Keep your hands in front of your elbows. Lower the bar slowly while keeping your elbows against your sides. Repeat for maximum repetitions.

Negative chin-up. In this exercise you'll do the positive phase of the chin-up with your legs and the negative phase with your arms. Using a chair or step for assistance, climb into the top position with your chin over the bar. Use an underhanded grip and space your hands shoulder-width apart. Remove your feet from the chair or step and lower your body slowly in 10 seconds. Quickly climb back to the top position with your chin over the bar. Repeat the slow lowering until you can no longer control your speed—which means the repetition will take only two to three seconds.

Wrist curl with barbell. Grasp a barbell with an underhanded grip. Rest your forearms on your thighs and the back of your hands against your knees and sit down. Lean forward until the angle between your upper arms and forearms is less than 90 degrees. Curl the bar smoothly and contract your forearm muscles. Pause. Lower the bar slowly and repeat.

Reverse wrist curl. Get in the same position as you did for the wrist curl except use an overhanded grip. Curl the bar upward smoothly. Do not move your forearms, shoulders, or torso forward or backward. Keep them stable. Lower the bar slowly. Repeat for maximum repetitions.

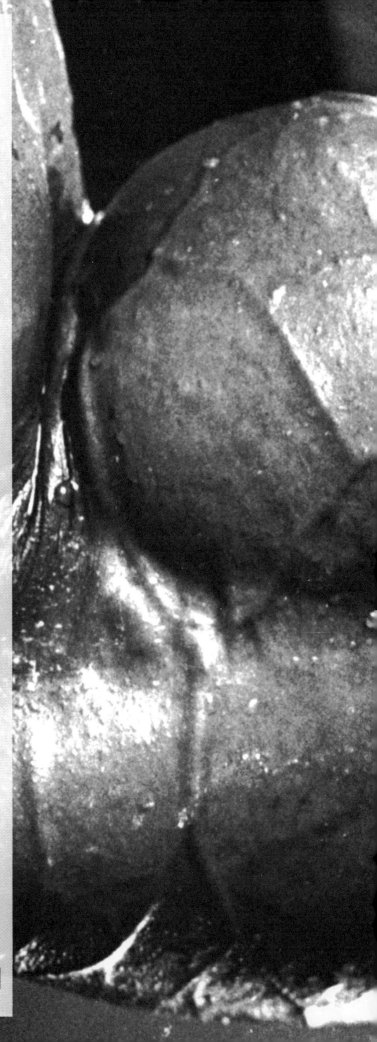

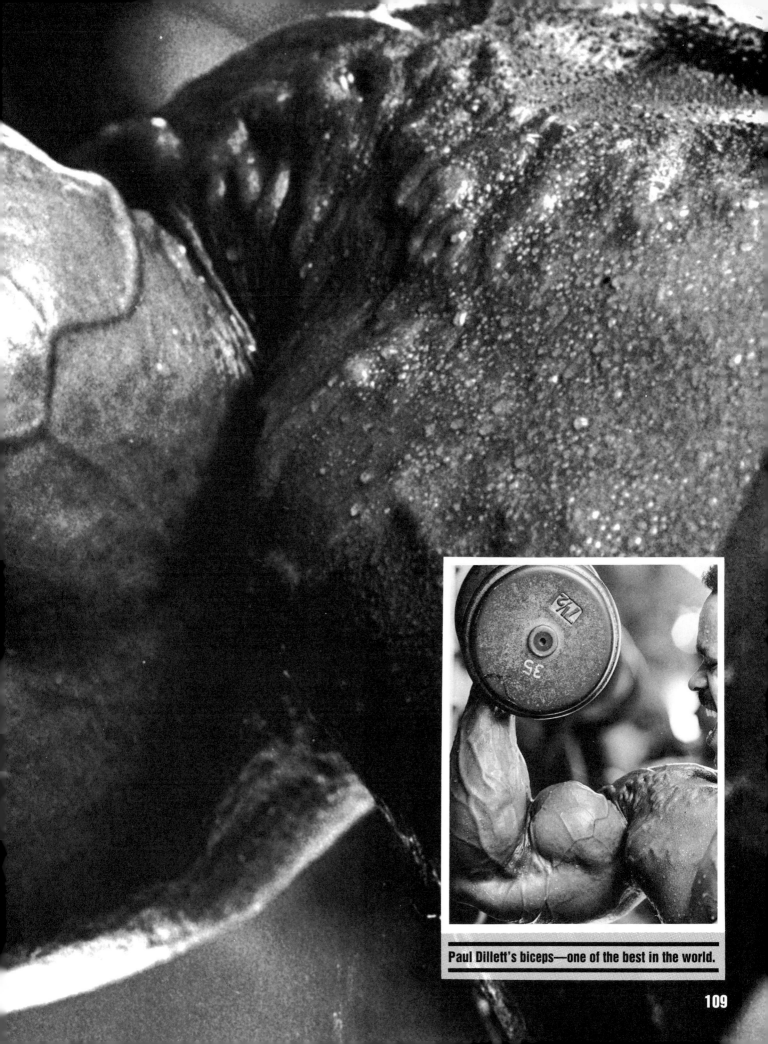

Paul Dillett's biceps—one of the best in the world.

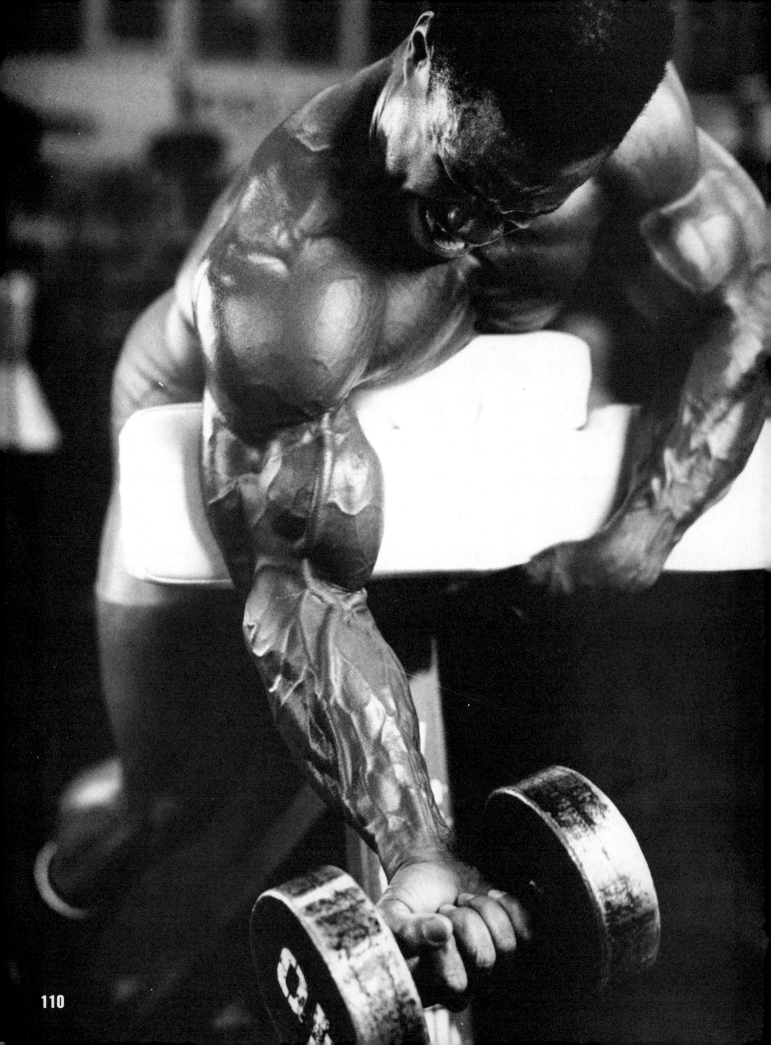

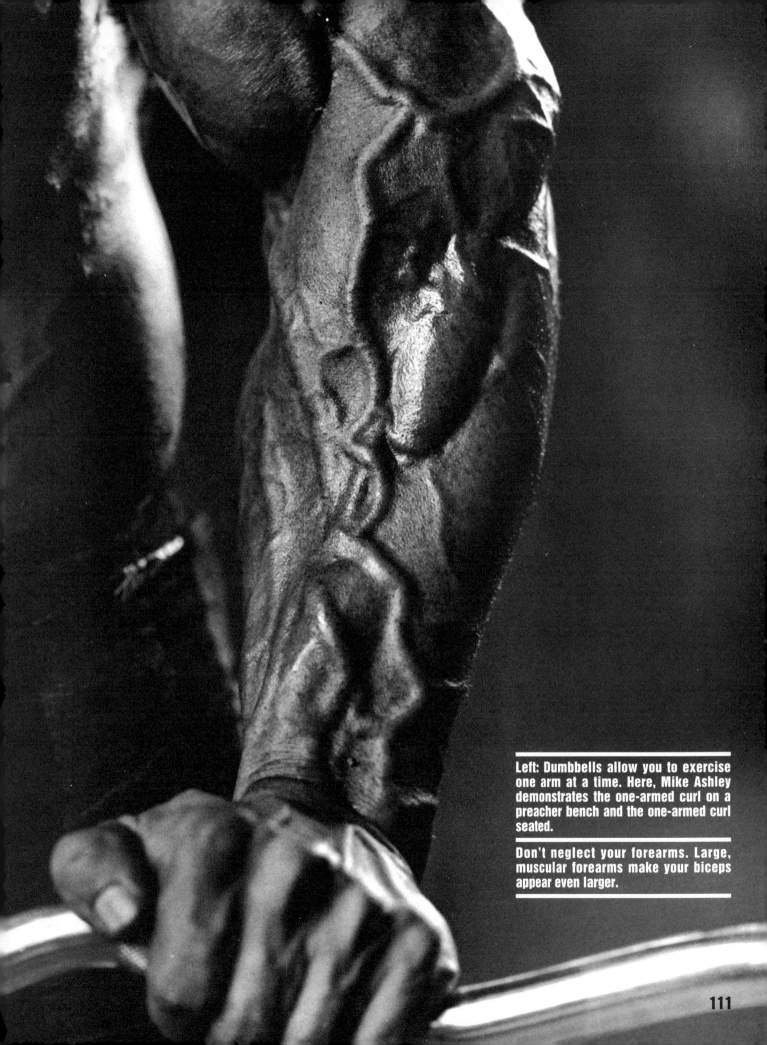

Left: Dumbbells allow you to exercise one arm at a time. Here, Mike Ashley demonstrates the one-armed curl on a preacher bench and the one-armed curl seated.

Don't neglect your forearms. Large, muscular forearms make your biceps appear even larger.

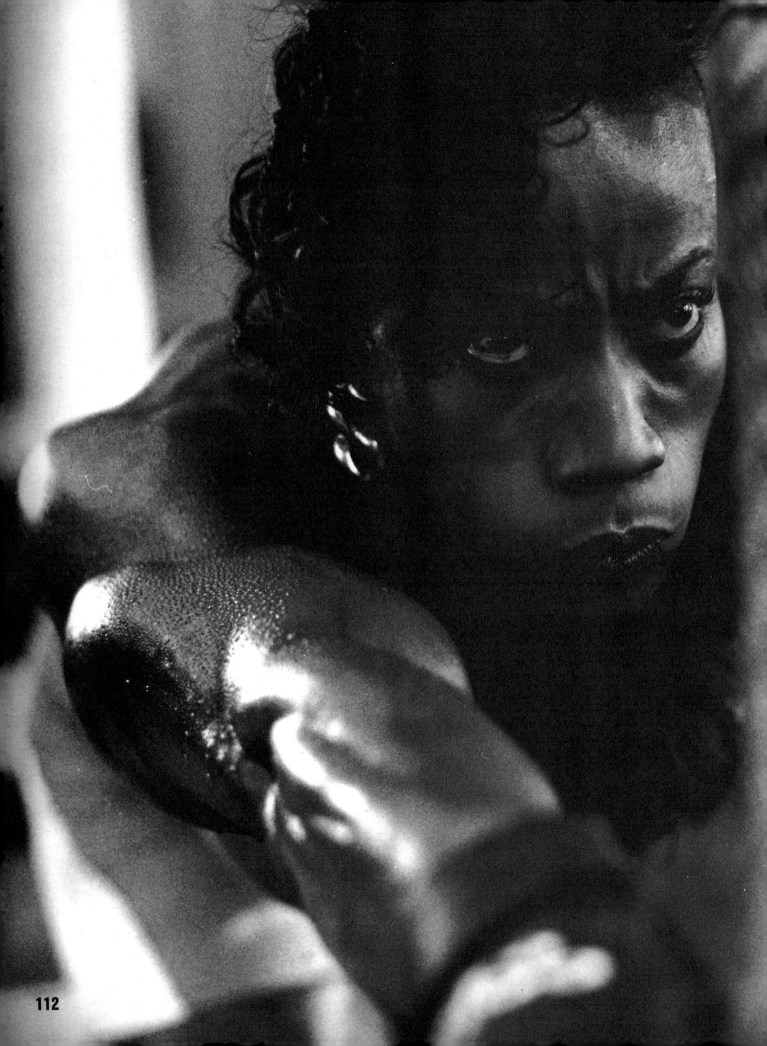

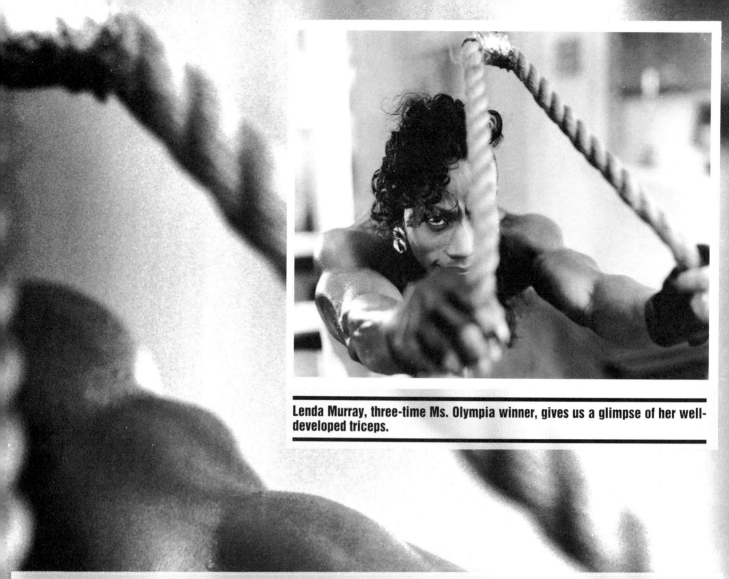

Lenda Murray, three-time Ms. Olympia winner, gives us a glimpse of her well-developed triceps.

26 • TRICEPS

The typical man's triceps, located on the back side of the upper arm, is from 25 to 50 percent larger than the typical biceps. If you really want massive arms, you must concentrate on your triceps.

Your triceps, like your biceps, crosses both your shoulder and elbow joints. The major function of the triceps is to extend the elbow. It also assists in bringing your upper arm down from an overhead position.

Here are three of the best triceps exercises:

<u>Triceps extension with one dumbbell</u>. Hold a single dumbbell on one end with both hands so that your palms are facing up, cradling the plates. Raise the dumbbell smoothly above your head. Keep your elbows tucked against the sides of your head and slowly lower the dumbbell behind your head until your forearms touch your biceps. Following the same path, raise the dumbbell overhead until your elbows are almost locked. Do as many repetitions as possible in good form.

<u>Dip</u>. Mount the parallel bars and straighten your arms. Stabilize yourself in the top position. Bend your arms and lower your body. Stretch comfortably at the bottom. Push smoothly back to the top while keeping your body momentum to a minimum. Repeat for maximum repetitions.

<u>Negative dip</u>. You'll probably require added resistance attached on a belt around your hips for the best results from negative dips. Place a sturdy chair or bench between the parallel bars. Climb into the top position. Remove your feet from the chair and stabilize your body. Bend your arms and lower your body slowly in 10 seconds. Stretch comfortably in the bottom. Climb back to the straight-arm position. Repeat this slow lowering until your speed going down is less than three seconds.

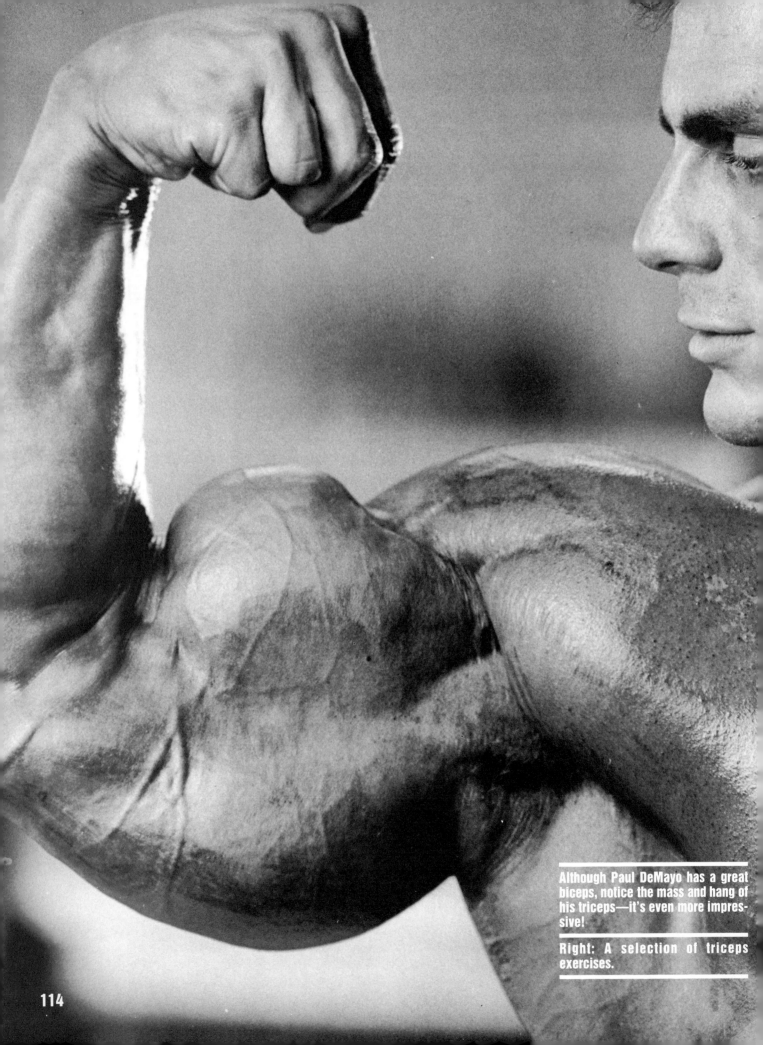

Although Paul DeMayo has a great biceps, notice the mass and hang of his triceps—it's even more impressive!

Right: A selection of triceps exercises.

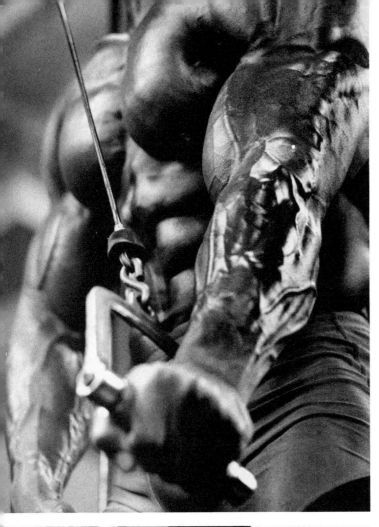
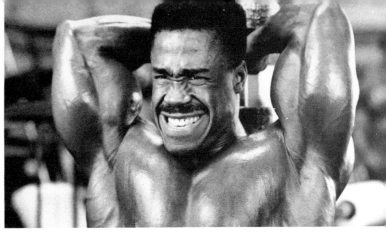
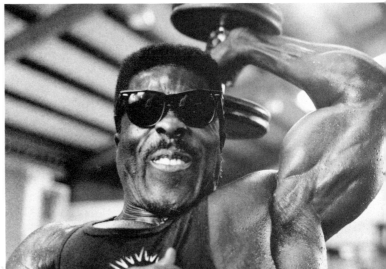
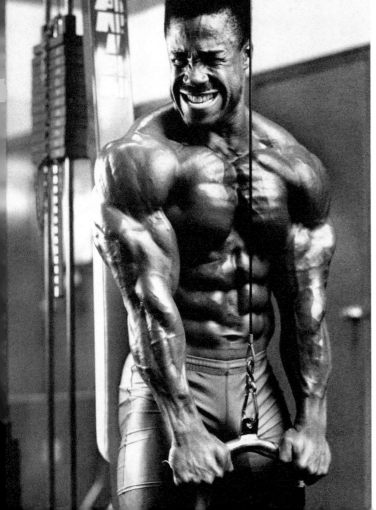
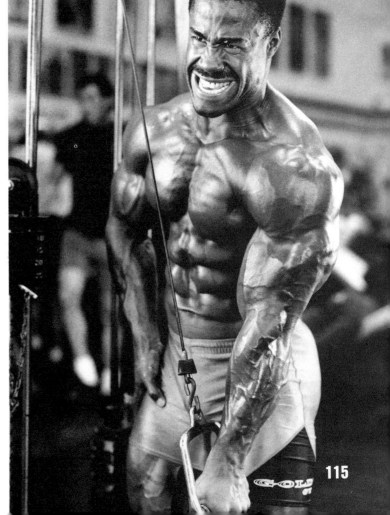

27 • ABDOMINALS

The most important muscle of your front waist is the rectus abdominis. Your rectus abdominis attaches to your ribs, extends down the front of your waist, and joins your pubis bone. When contracted the rectus abdominis moves your ribs closer to your navel.

Underneath the rectus abdominis is the iliopsoas muscles. When the iliopsoas muscles contract they pull your upper body to a sitting position, or they move your thighs toward your chest.

The bent-kneed sit-up involves both the rectus abdominis and iliopsoas muscles. The reverse trunk curl isolates the rectus abdominis. Here's the best way to perform each one:

Bent-kneed sit-up. A high sit-up board works well for this exercise. With your knees bent at a 90-degree angle, hook your feet under the roller pads at the top. Lie on your back and position your hands behind your head. Curl your shoulders first, then your torso, and touch your chest to your thighs. Lower your torso and shoulders slowly back to the starting position. Do as many smooth repetitions as you can.

Reverse trunk curl. This exercise zeros in on the muscles behind your navel. Lie face up on the floor with your hands on either side of your hips. Bring your thighs to your chest so your knees and hips are in a flexed position. Curl your hips toward your chest smoothly by lifting your buttocks and lower back off the floor. At the same time that you lift your buttocks, you must counterbalance your body by pushing down on the floor with your hands and arms. Pause briefly in the top position. Lower your hips slowly to the floor. Repeat for maximum repetitions.

Proper eating and proper exercising are responsible for the award-winning midsection of Thierry Pastel.

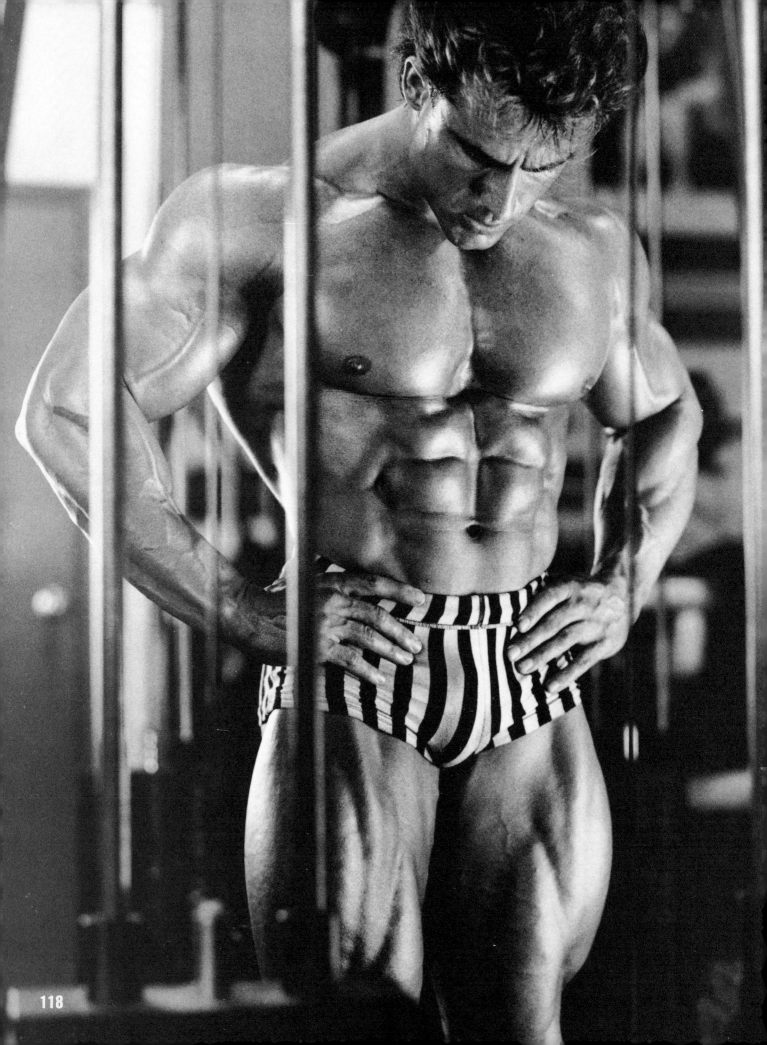

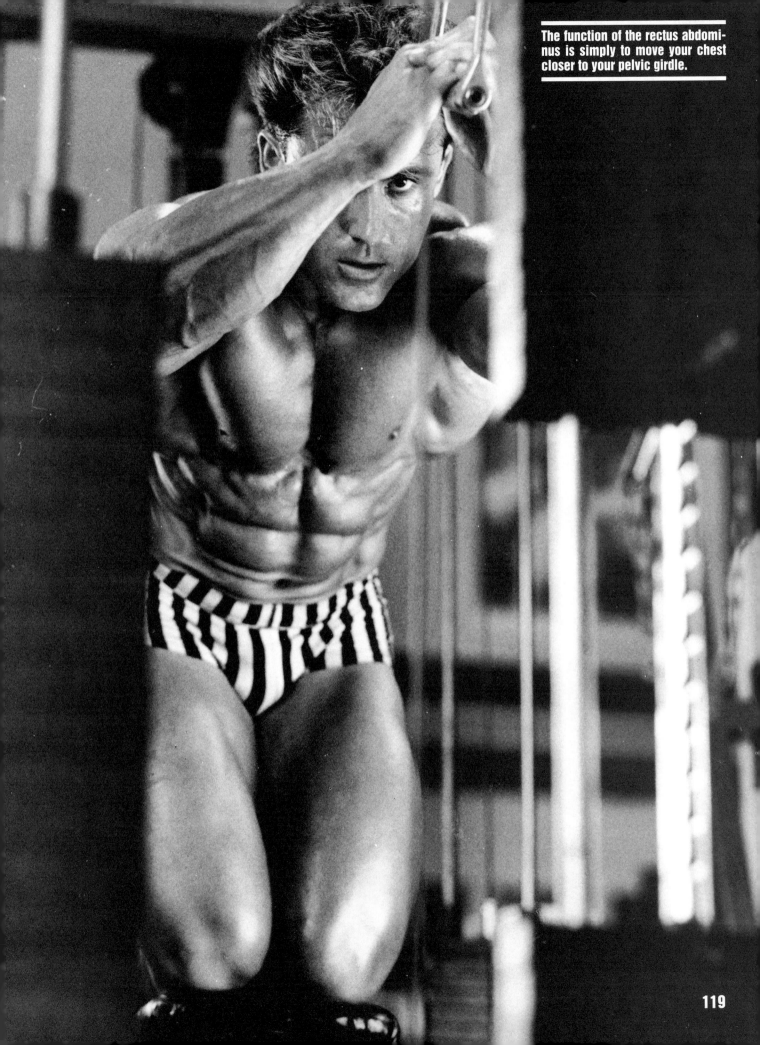

The function of the rectus abdominus is simply to move your chest closer to your pelvic girdle.

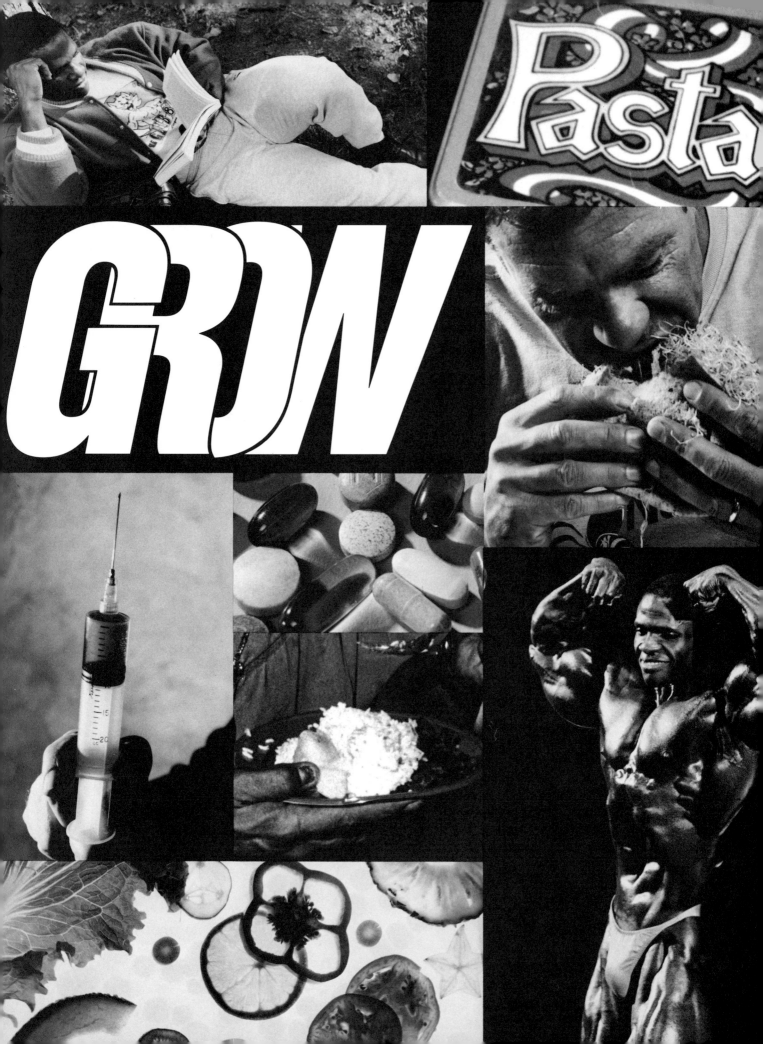

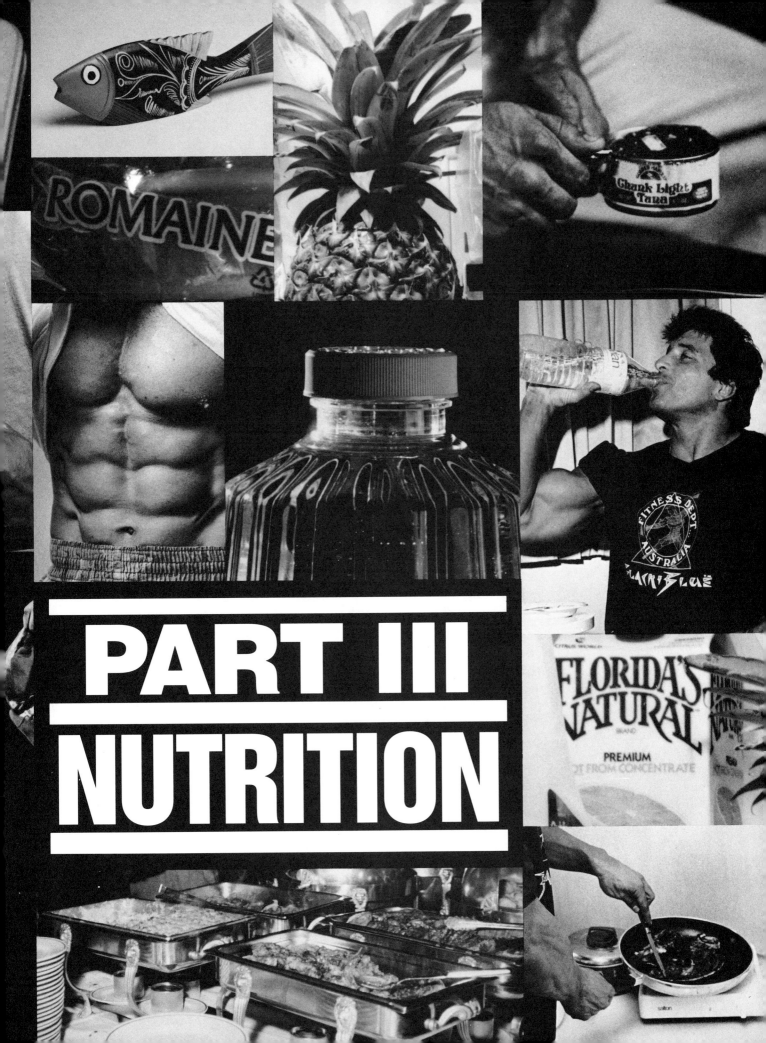

PART III
NUTRITION

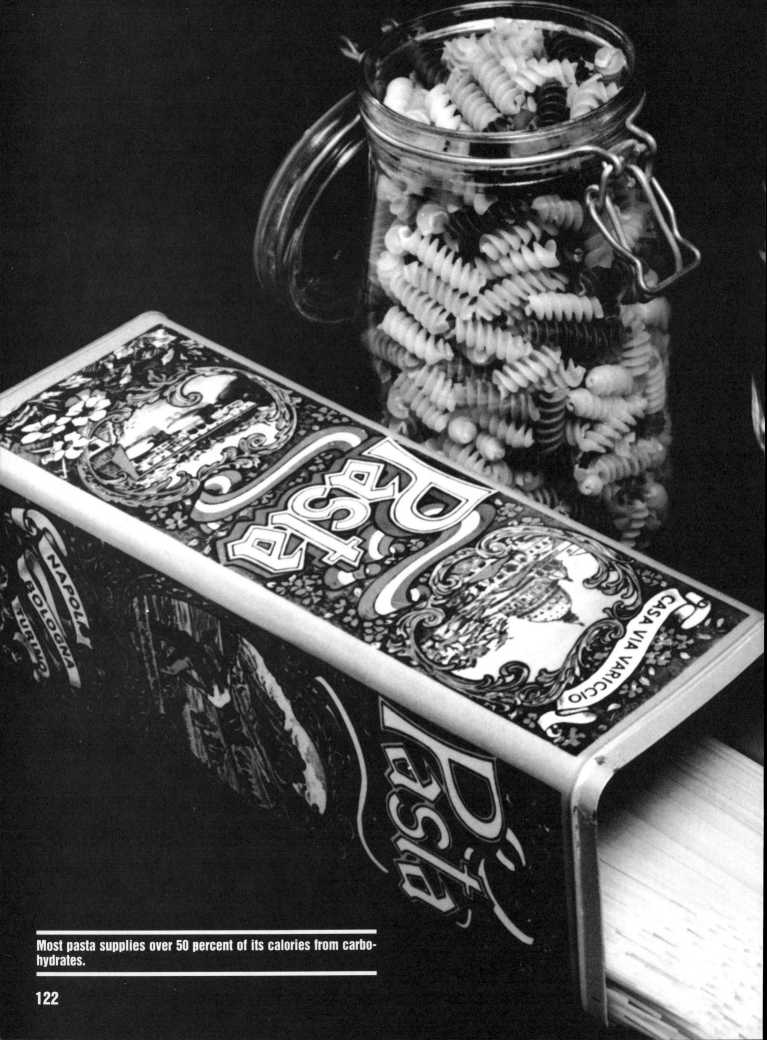

Most pasta supplies over 50 percent of its calories from carbo-hydrates.

28 • CARBOHYDRATES

Carbohydrate is the term used to describe the class of foods commonly known as sugars and starches. All carbohydrates are composed of carbon, hydrogen, and oxygen.

The eating plan that worked so well for Jeff Turner, which is described in Part IV, was made up of a daily breakdown of 60 percent carbohydrates, 15 percent proteins, and 25 percent fats. A carbohydrate-rich diet is necessary for maximum muscle growth.

Recommended carbohydrate-rich foods are as follows:

Potatoes	Fruits	Beans	Breads	Lentils
Corn	Rice	Cereals	Peas	Pasta

The primary functions of carbohydrates in the body are to provide an economical energy supply, to furnish important vitamins and minerals as well as some proteins, to supply fiber, and to add flavor to foods and beverages.

Remember, 60 percent of your calories each day should come from carbohydrates.

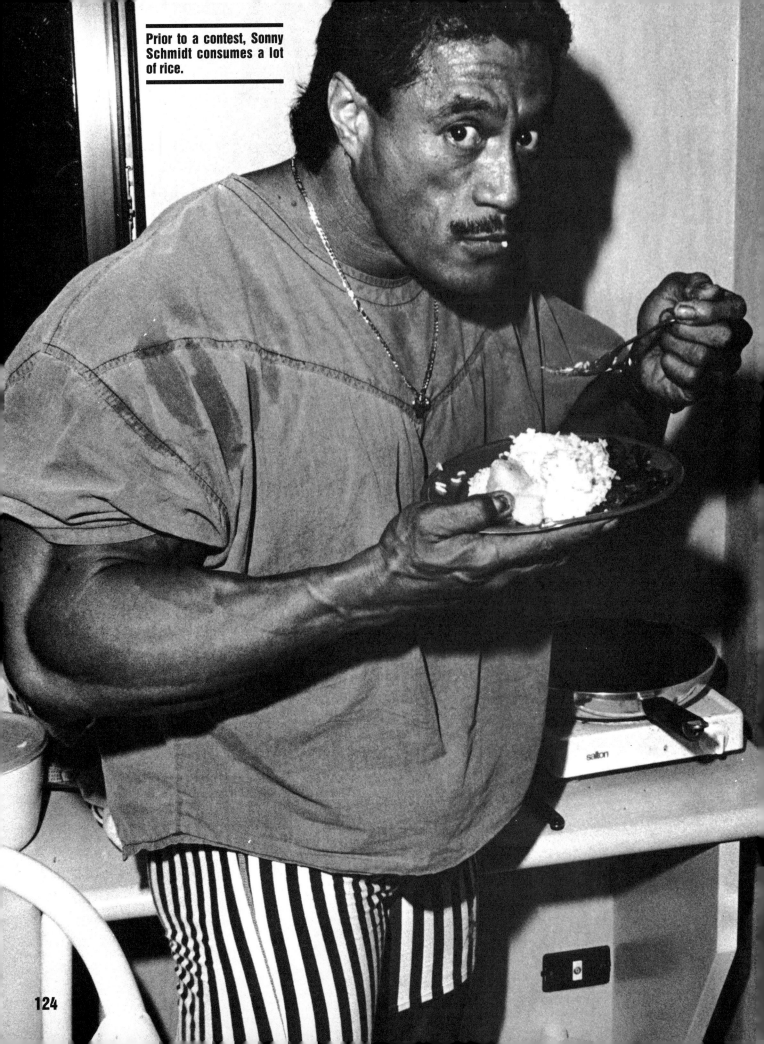

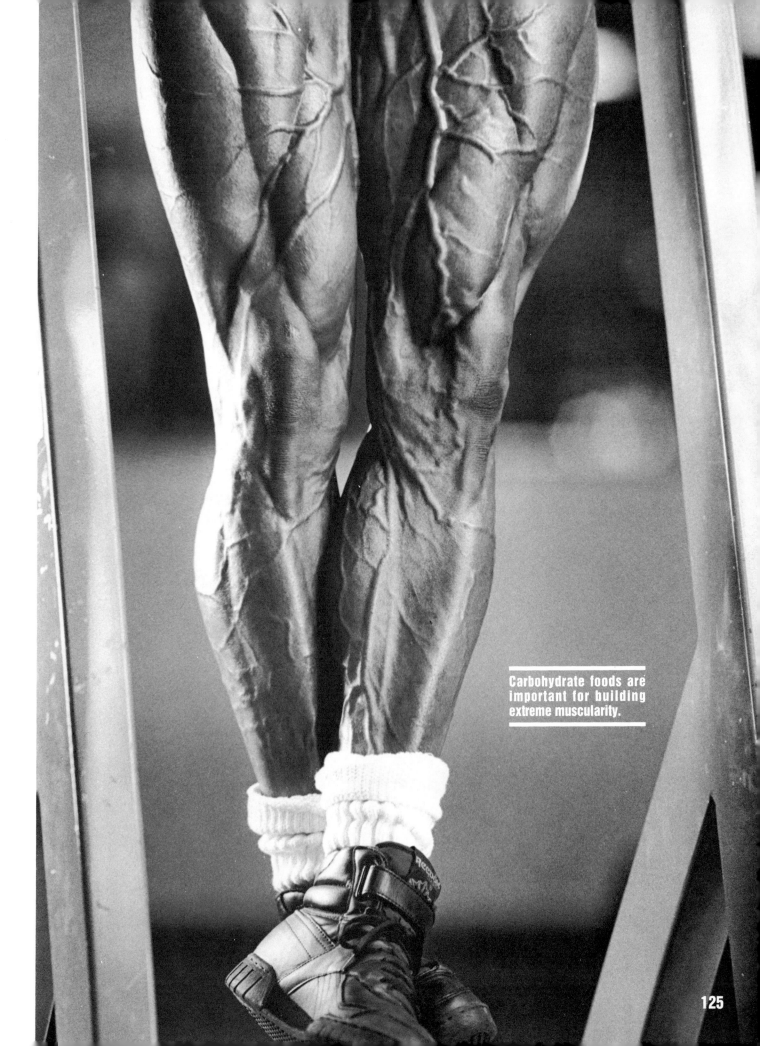

Carbohydrate foods are important for building extreme muscularity.

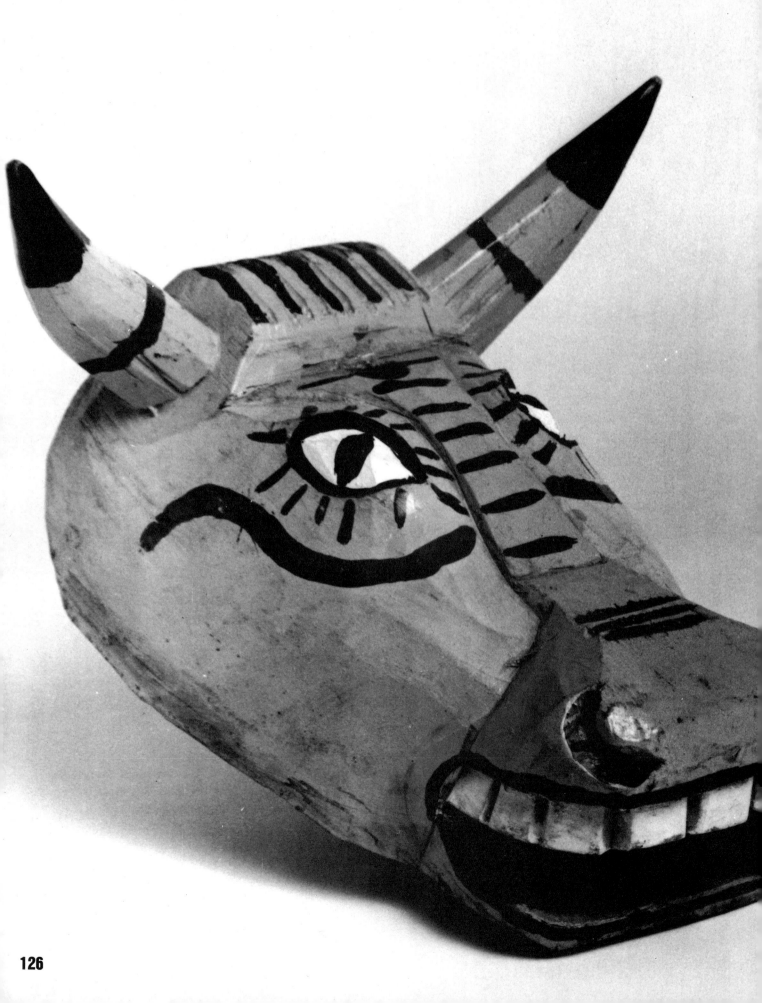

29 • PROTEINS

Traditionally, bodybuilders have always devoured plenty of protein foods, such as chicken, beef, fish, eggs, and milk. The theory was that if you consumed a lot of protein, you'd build huge muscles.

Research has repeatedly shown that extra protein does not cause your muscles to grow. Exercise, not protein, is the most important factor. Nevertheless, you certainly do not want to de-emphasize protein.

Protein is composed of carbon, hydrogen, and oxygen—but in addition it contains nitrogen. These atoms are arranged into amino acids, which are used as building blocks throughout your body.

If you examine the scientific literature concerning dietary protein, you'll find that several facts emerge:

- The average person (including the athlete) in the United States is not lacking in protein. In fact, he or she consumes well over the Recommended Dietary Allowance of protein each day.
- Intense bodybuilding exercise does not significantly increase an athlete's requirement for protein.
- There are no significant nutritional benefits from the use of protein supplements, including the latest free-form amino acids.
- Excessive amounts of protein, including concentrated supplements, can cause damage to the liver and kidneys.
- The Recommended Dietary Allowance for protein is .36 grams per pound of body weight. This is an excellent guideline for bodybuilders to follow.
- The guidelines and menus in Part IV, which call for 15 percent of your daily calories to be from protein-rich foods, provides more than ample protein for maximum growth.

Examples of protein-rich foods are as follows:

Lean Meats   Cheese   Beans   Poultry   Yogurt
Skim milk   Lentils Fish   Nuts   Tofu

For better bodybuilding results, consume protein foods in moderation.

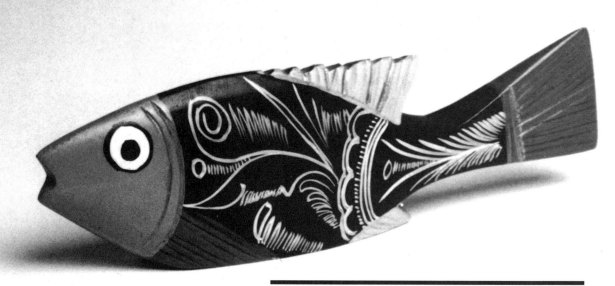

Beef and fish are rich sources of the essential amino acids.

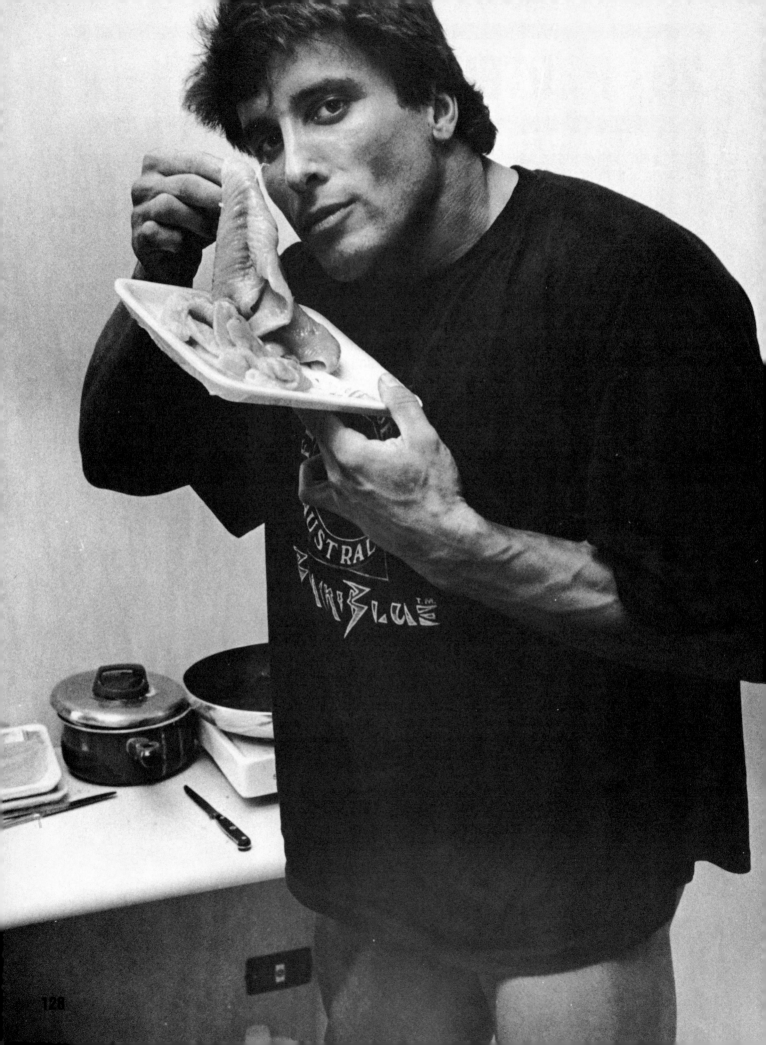

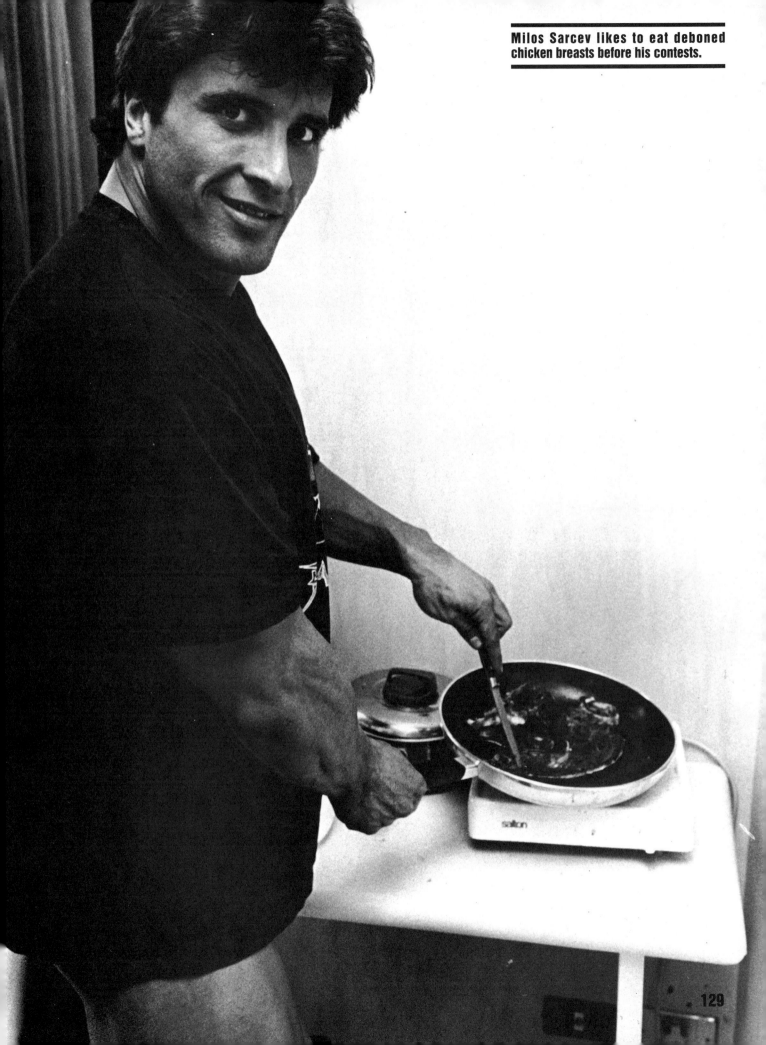

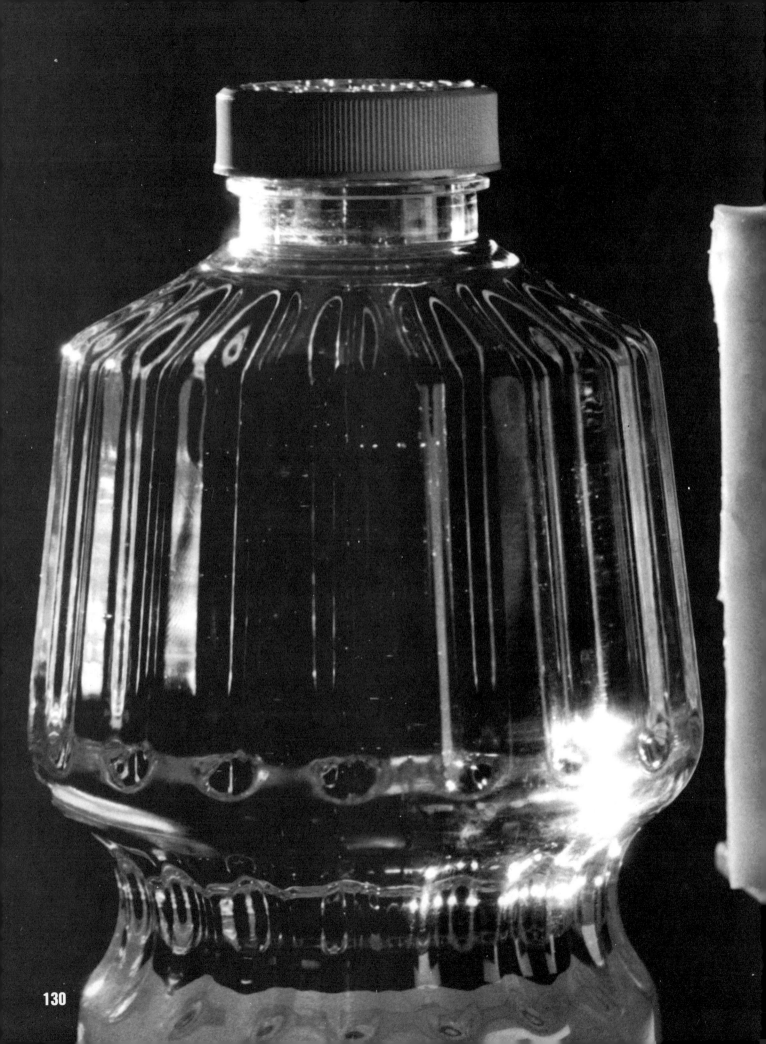

30 • FATS

Many people believe that the less fat you have on your body, and the less fat you eat, the better. This is not correct. Like all nutrients, fat is beneficial in appropriate amounts, and it is harmful to consume too much or too little.

Gram for gram, fats provide 2.25 times as much energy or calories as either carbohydrates or proteins. They also carry the fat-soluble vitamins A, D, E, and K. Fats perform the following functions:

- They compose part of the structure of cells.
- They spare protein for growth and repair by providing energy.
- They supply important satiety value to food.
- They make foods appetizing and flavorful.
- They provide linoleic acid—an essential fatty acid.

Approximately 20 to 25 percent of your daily calories should come from fats. The menus presented in Part IV are composed of 25 percent fats. Examine them closely.

Oil and cheese contain concentrated fat calories, which you should consume in moderation.

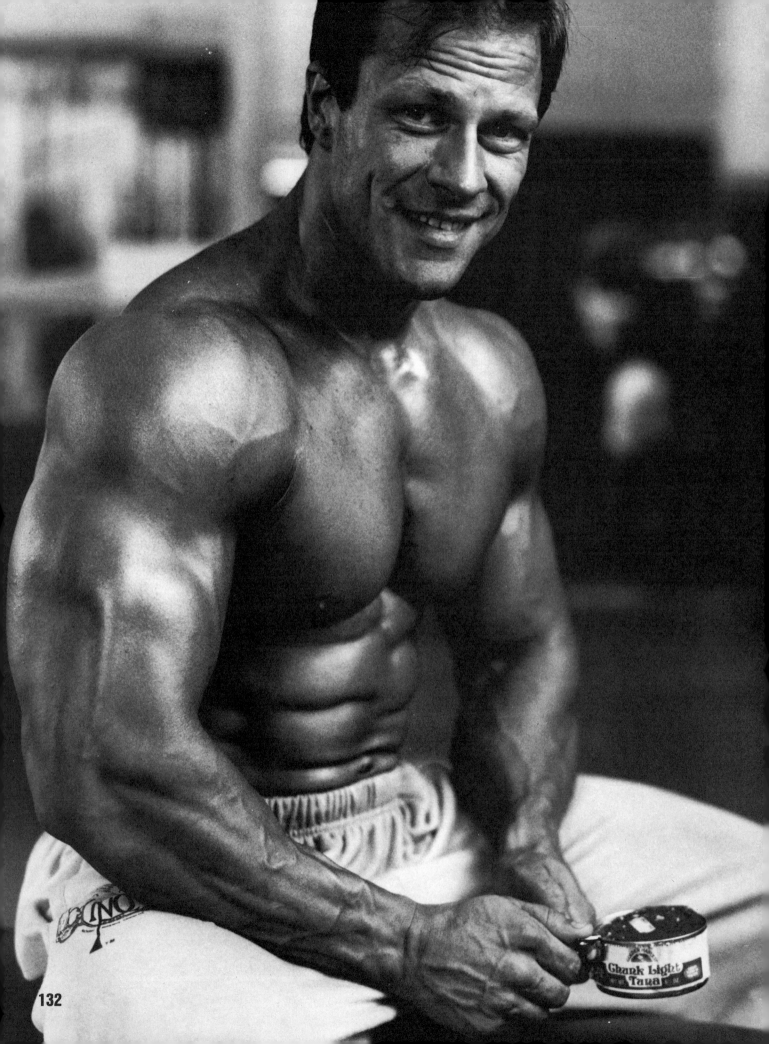

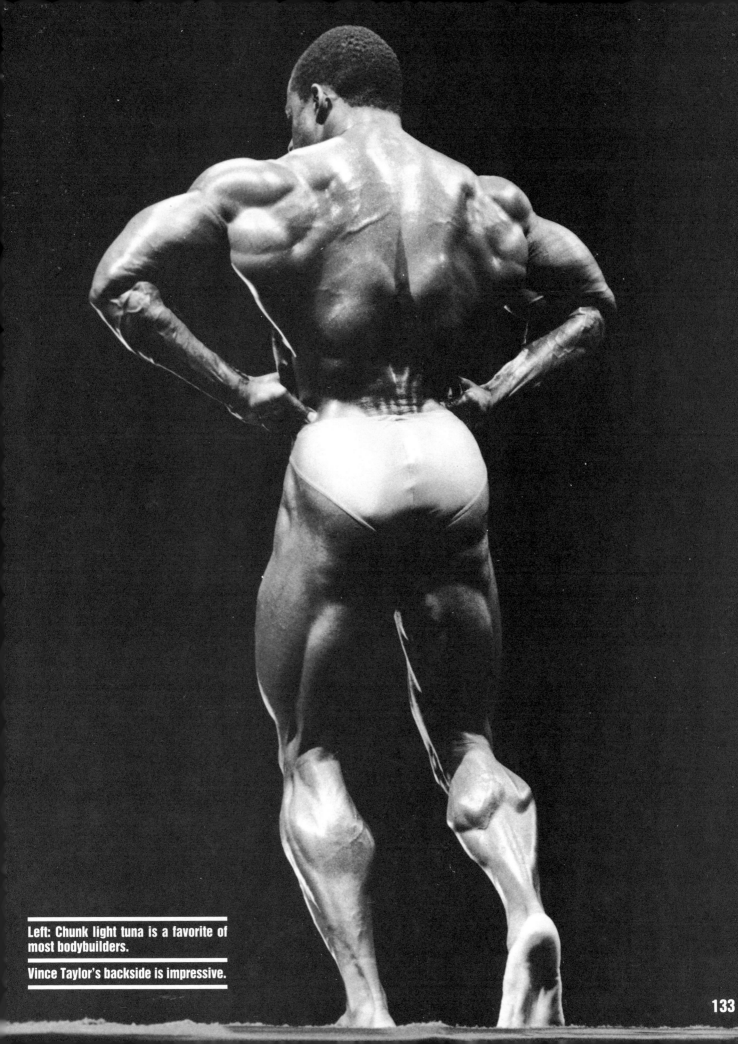

Left: Chunk light tuna is a favorite of most bodybuilders.

Vince Taylor's backside is impressive.

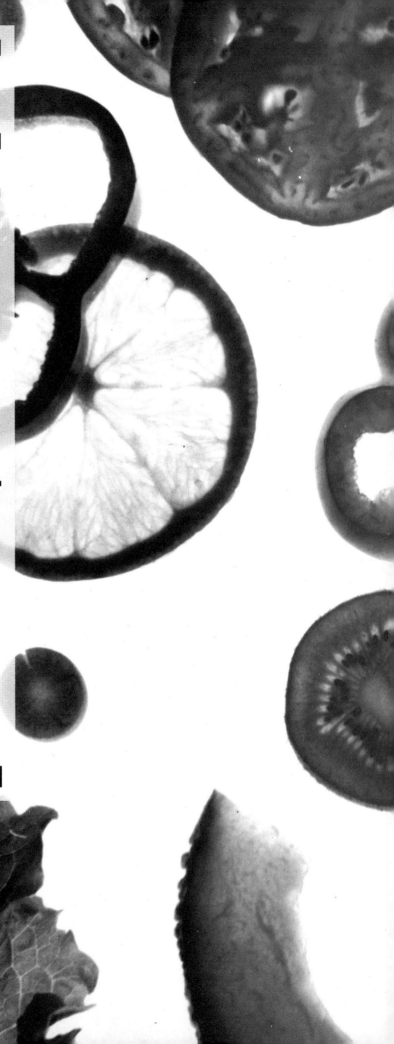

31 • VITAMINS

Vitamins are potent, noncaloric compounds needed in very small amounts in your diet. They perform specific functions to promote growth and reproduction or to maintain health and life.

This description separates the vitamins from carbohydrates, proteins, and fats. Unlike these nutrients, vitamins do not provide calories or energy.

To date, 13 vitamins have been discovered, each with a specific purpose. For example, vitamin A is part of an eye pigment that helps you see in dim light, vitamin B_1 helps convert glucose into energy, and vitamin D controls the way your body uses calcium.

Vitamins are categorized according to whether they are soluble in fat or water.

Fat-Soluble Vitamins	Water-Soluble Vitamins
Vitamin A	Ascorbic acid (Vitamin C)
Vitamin D	B-Complex Vitamins
Vitamin E	Thiamin (Vitamin B_1)
Vitamin K	Riboflavin (Vitamin B_2)
	Pyridoxine (Vitamin B_6)
	Nicotinic acid (Niacin)
	Pantothenic acid
	Folic acid
	Vitamin B_{12}
	Biotin

All of these vitamins occur widely in many foods and are easily provided in a mixed diet containing fresh fruits and vegetables and whole grains.

Fruits and vegetables have been called the "original health foods," since they are loaded with vitamins.

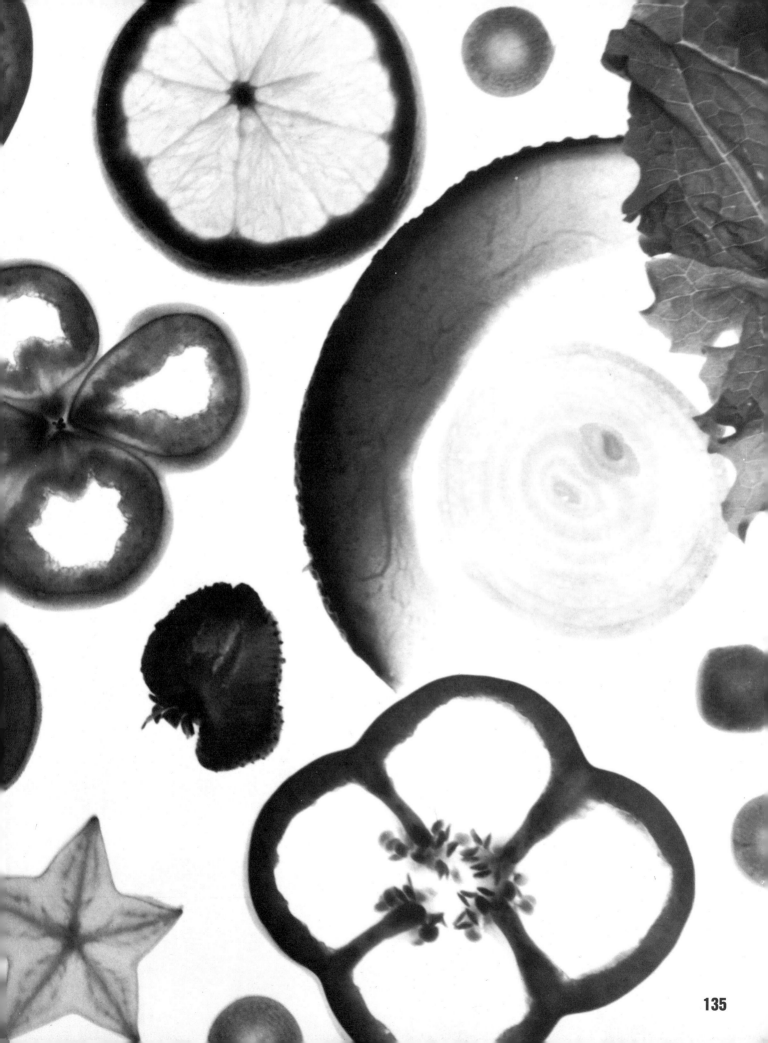

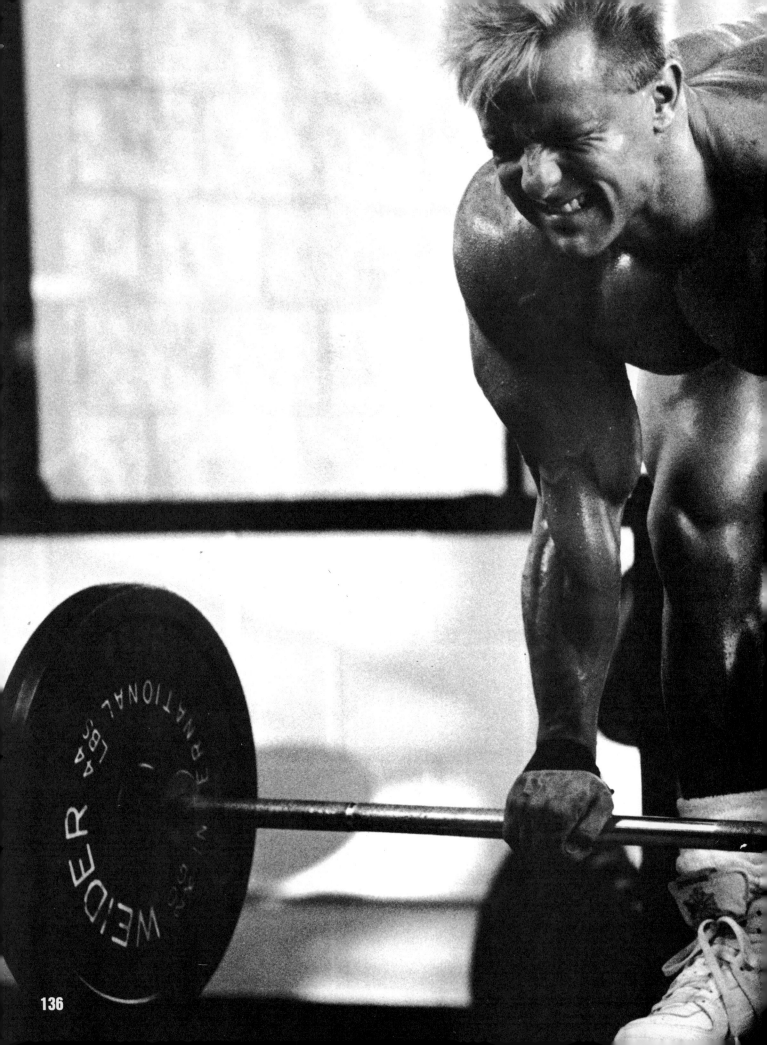

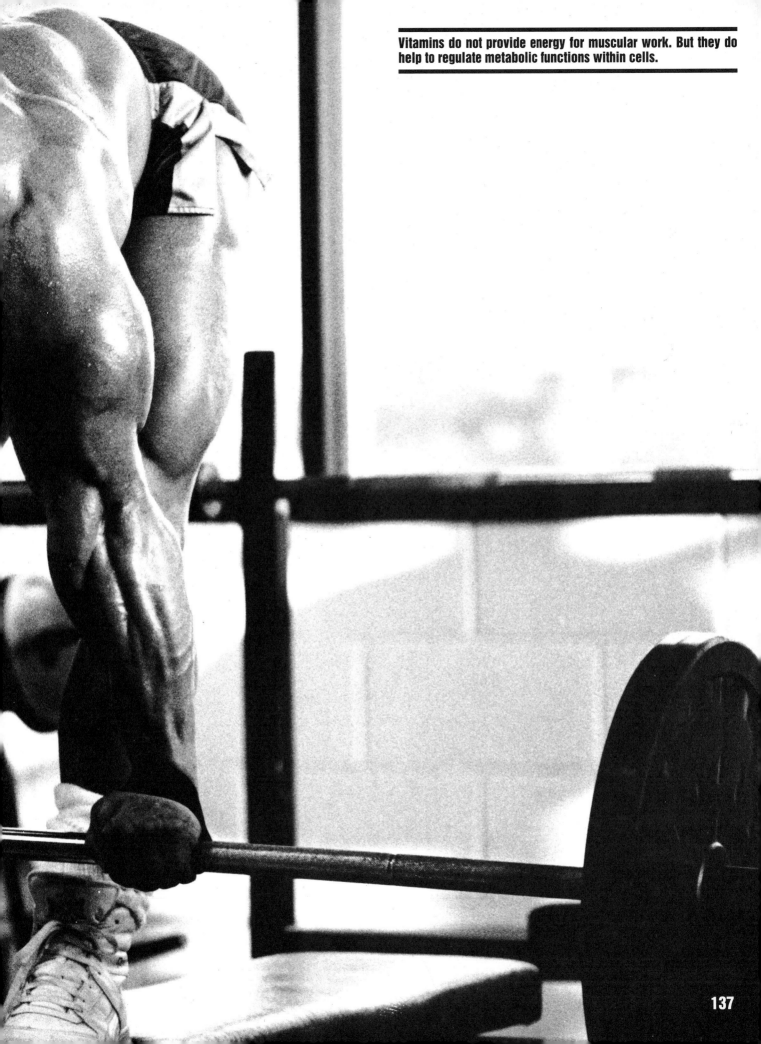

32 • MINERALS

Minerals occur freely in nature in the soil and water. They travel through the food chain by being absorbed into the plants that grow in the soil and then into the animals that consume the plants and water.

Unlike vitamins, minerals tend to be incorporated into the actual structures and working chemicals of your body. Vitamins function mainly as catalysts. They promote chemical processes without actually becoming part of the products of the reactions. Minerals become involved in the building of enzymes and actual tissue structures.

Each mineral has a unique role in your body. For example, calcium provides the rigid structure of the bones, potassium and sodium control water balance in your body, iron assists with oxygen transport, and magnesium activates enzymes and is required for muscle contraction.

You need some minerals in only trace amounts: iron, zinc, selenium, and iodine. Others—such as calcium, potassium, sodium, chloride, phosphorus, and magnesium—are needed in greater amounts.

As with vitamins, you can get all the minerals you need if you consume a variety of wholesome foods each day. Chapter 34 shows you how to do this in a fail-safe manner.

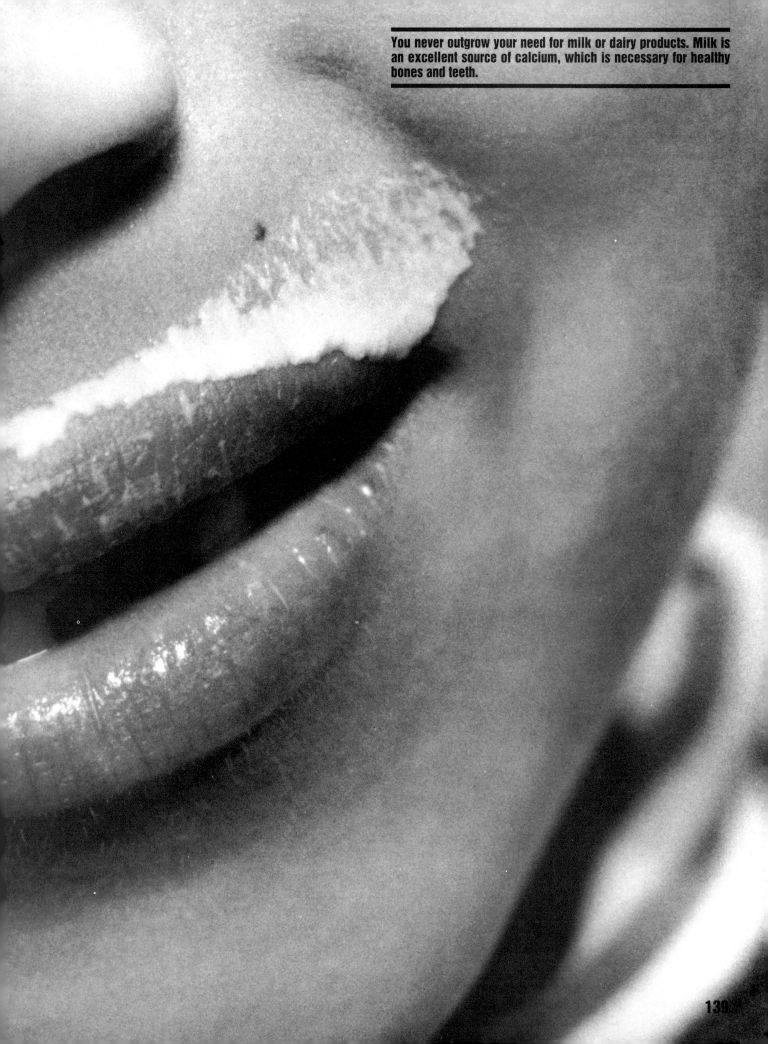

You never outgrow your need for milk or dairy products. Milk is an excellent source of calcium, which is necessary for healthy bones and teeth.

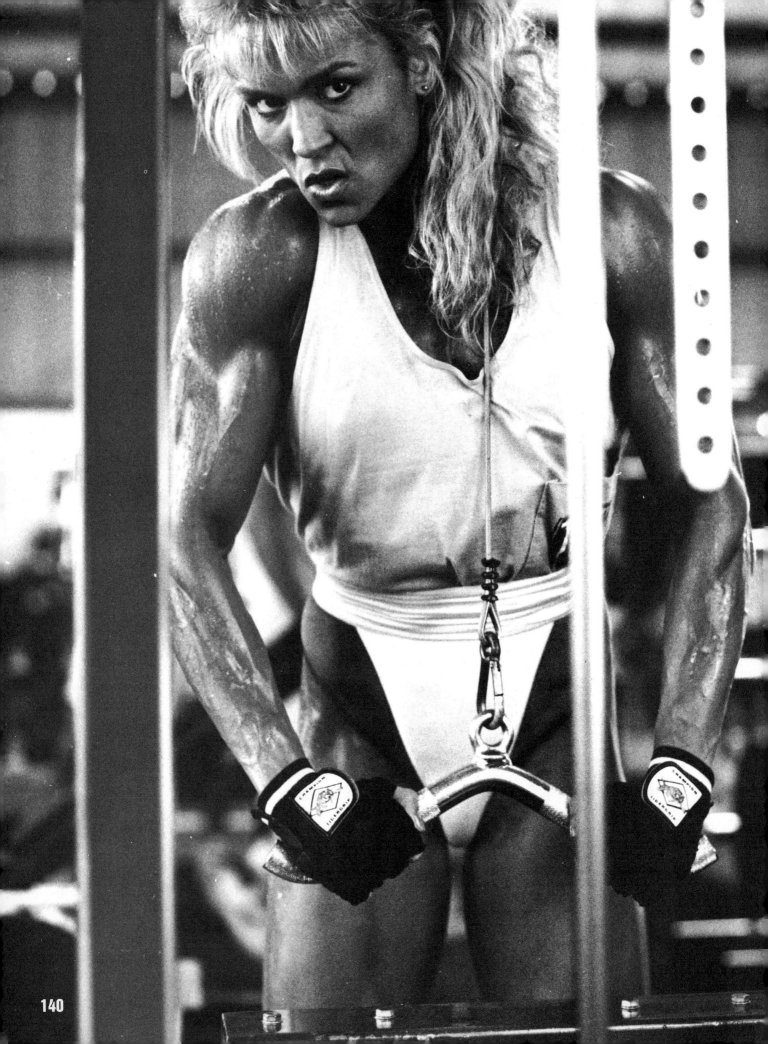

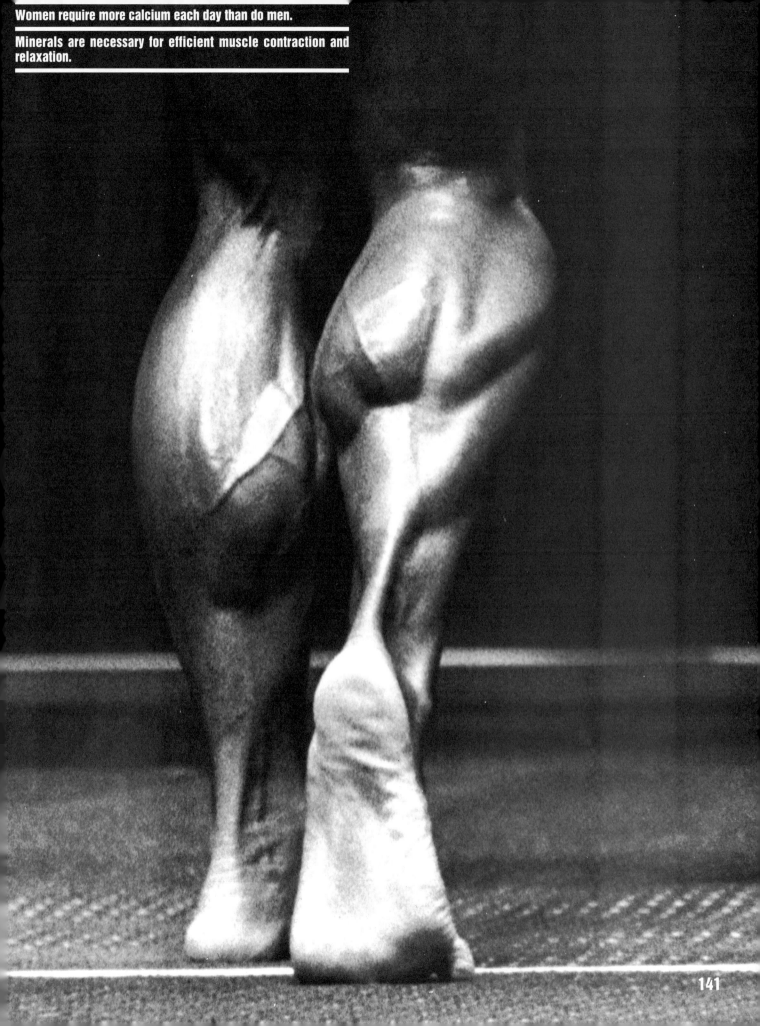

33 • WATER

Water is a simple compound composed of two hydrogen atoms and one oxygen atom (H_2O).

Water is just as important to good nutrition as are carbohydrates, proteins, fats, vitamins, and minerals. Unfortunately, many bodybuilders do not realize this.

In your body, water functions as a building material, solvent, lubricant, and temperature regulator. It serves as a building material in the construction of every cell. The water content of cells varies; for example, the water content of teeth is less than 10 percent: bones, 25 percent; and muscle, 70 percent.

As a solvent, water is used in the digestive processes by aiding in the chewing and softening of food. It also supplies fluid for your digestive juices and facilitates movement of the food mass along your digestive tract. After digestion, water as blood is the means by which nutrients are carried to your cells and waste products are removed.

Water also serves as a lubricant in your joints and between your internal organs. It keeps your cells moist and permits the passage of substances between your cells and blood vessels. Water also serves the very important function of removing heat from your body by its evaporation as sweat.

How much water should you drink each day? My recommendation for bodybuilders is to consume one gallon, or 128 ounces, each 24 hours. This can be easily accomplished if you carry a bottle of water—one of those quart-size insulated containers with a plastic straw, for example—and sip from it all day long.

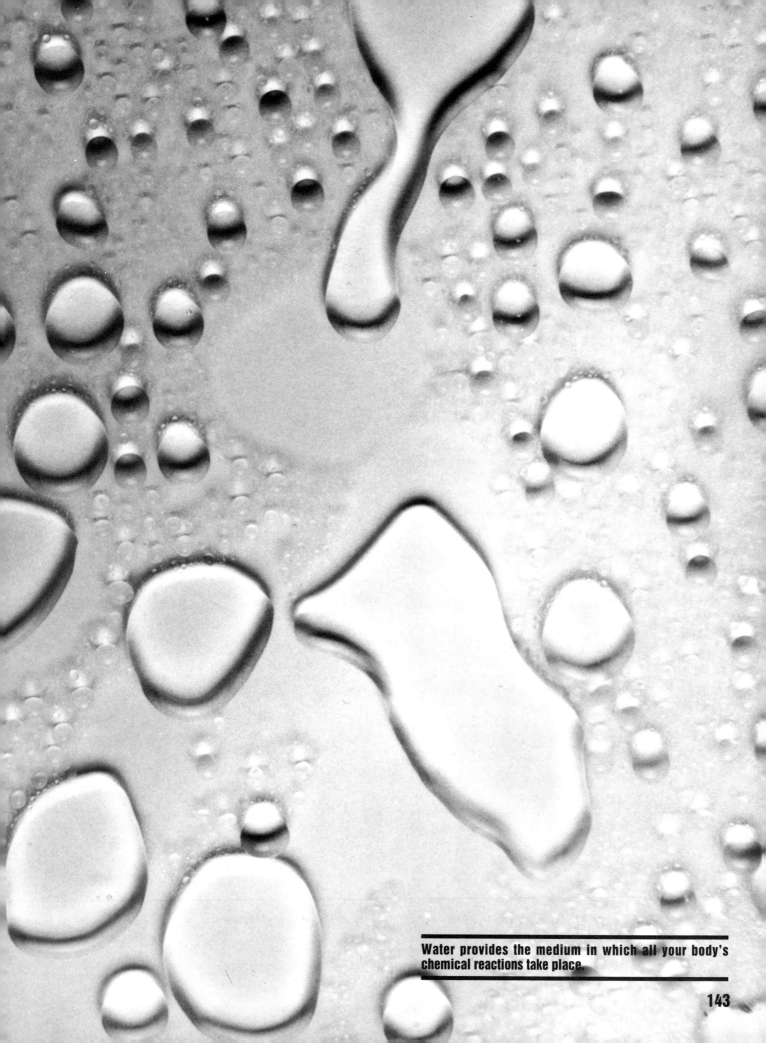

Water provides the medium in which all your body's chemical reactions take place.

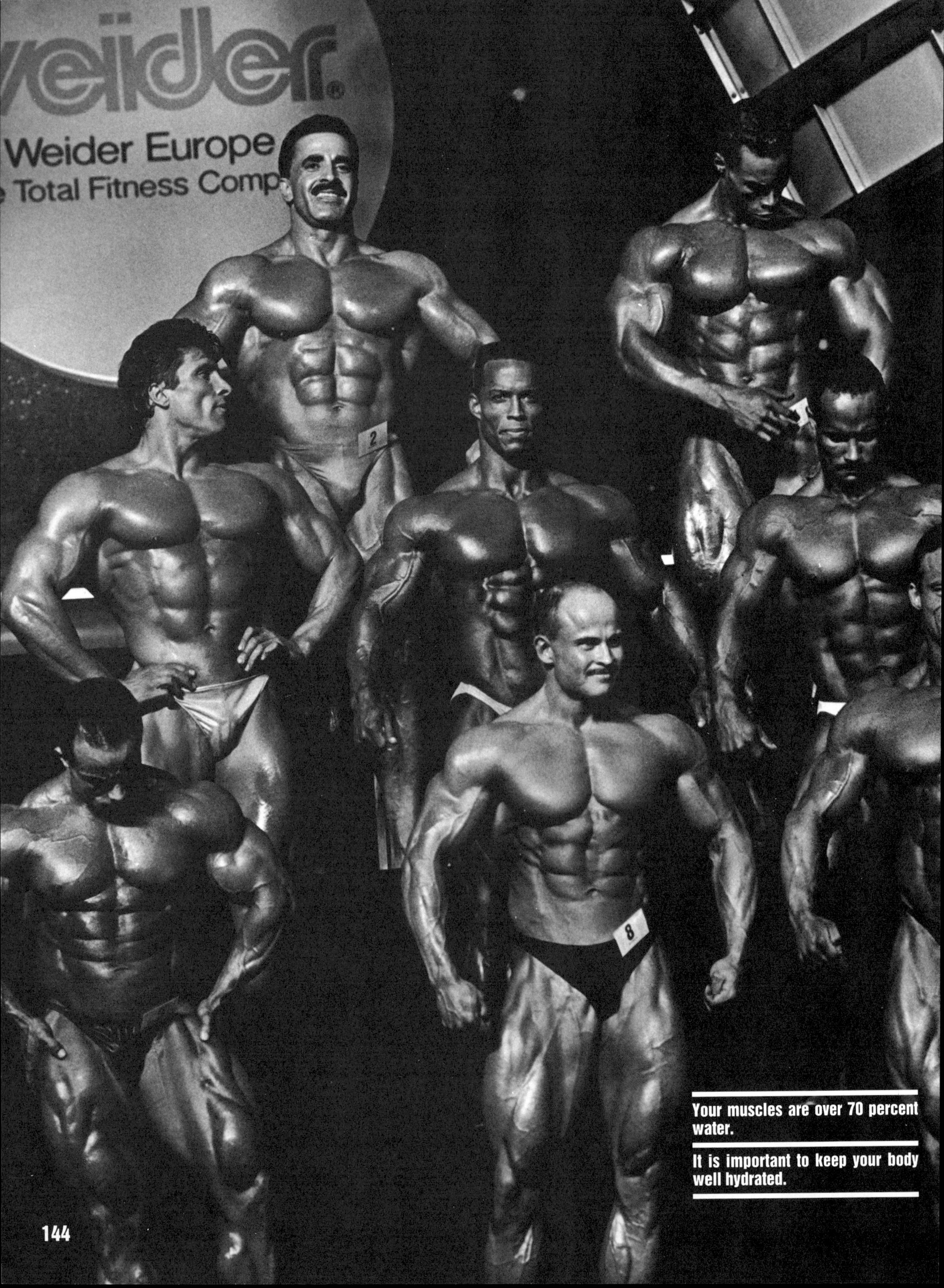

Your muscles are over 70 percent water.

It is important to keep your body well hydrated.

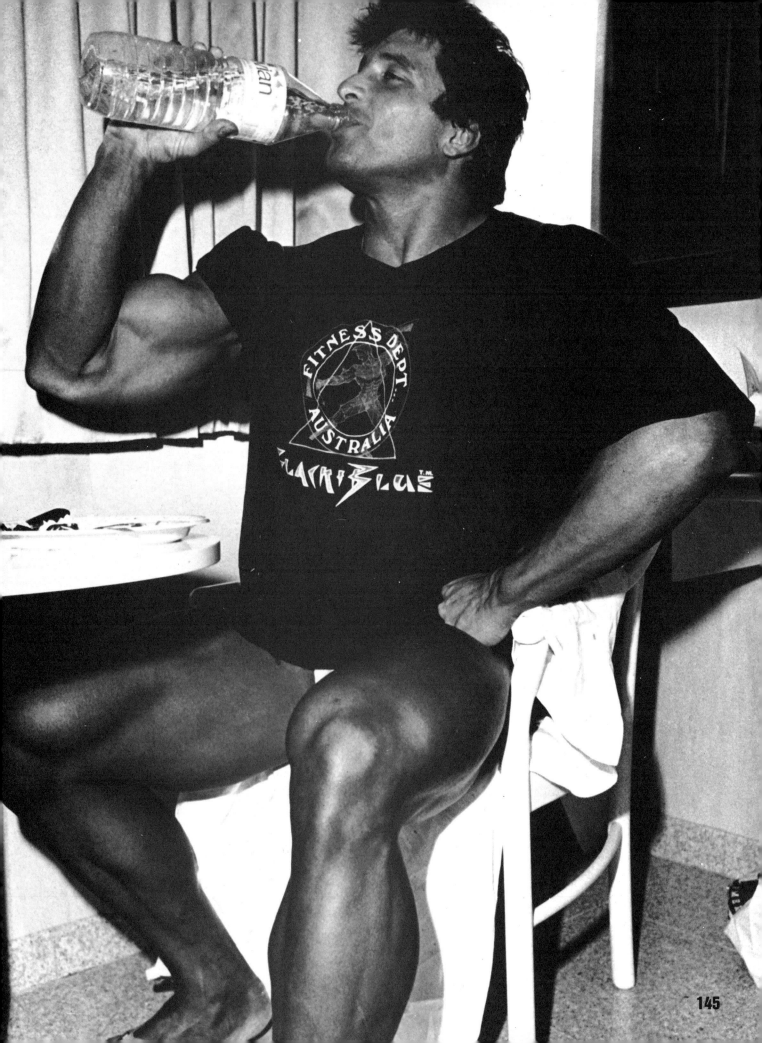

34 • MEALS

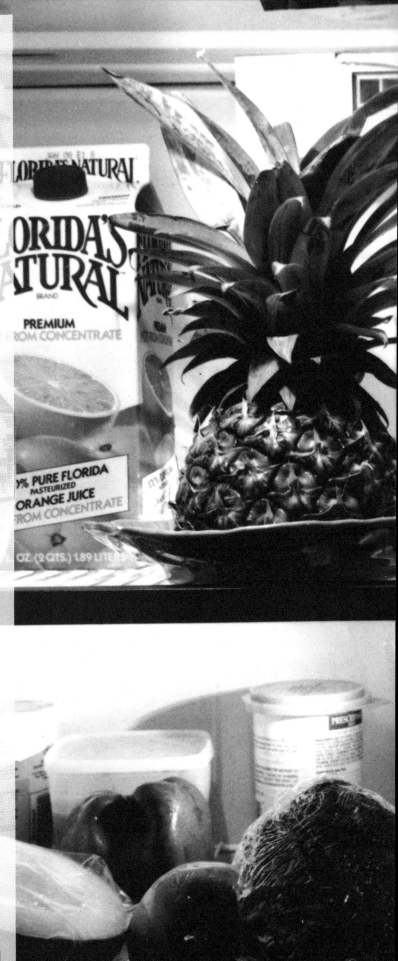

Fifty years ago the U.S. Department of Agriculture devised a plan for well-balanced eating, consisting of seven food groups. In 1958 these recommendations were simplified to four food groups. Two to four servings from the Basic Four—meat, milk, fruits and vegetables, and breads and cereals—on a daily basis was considered to be well-balanced eating.

I've successfully applied the Basic Four to bodybuilding for over 20 years. It's always worked well for me and my trainees.

Recently, the Basic Four has been criticized as leading to meals that were too high in fats and proteins and too low in carbohydrates. As a result, in 1992 the Department of Agriculture expanded the Basic Four to six food groups, which closely resemble the seven food groups of the 1940s.

In my experience, however, what's needed is a better appreciation of the Basic Four. When applied correctly, the Basic Four food groups can work very well for the bodybuilder who desires to grow.

The general eating plan for one day translates to:

- four servings from the meat/poultry/fish/ legumes/egg group
- four servings from the milk/yogurt/cheese group
- eight servings from the fruit/vegetable group
- eight servings from the bread/cereal group

The above serving ratio of 4:4:8:8 yields a diet of approximately 55 to 65 percent carbohydrates, 20 to 25 percent fats, and 15 to 20 percent proteins. This is an ideal breakdown for bodybuilding.

For the last two years I've worked with Stacey Goss, one of the owners of Computerized Bodyweight Management Systems in Colorado Springs. Stacey has a unique way of separating foods into more than 20 groups; then she has you select the foods you like best from each group and organizes a specific eating plan based on your selections.

In Part IV, I'll detail how Stacey organized the 28-day eating plan for Jeff Turner. Furthermore, I'll show you how you can do something similar with your meals.

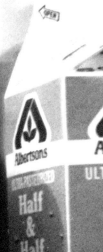
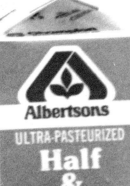

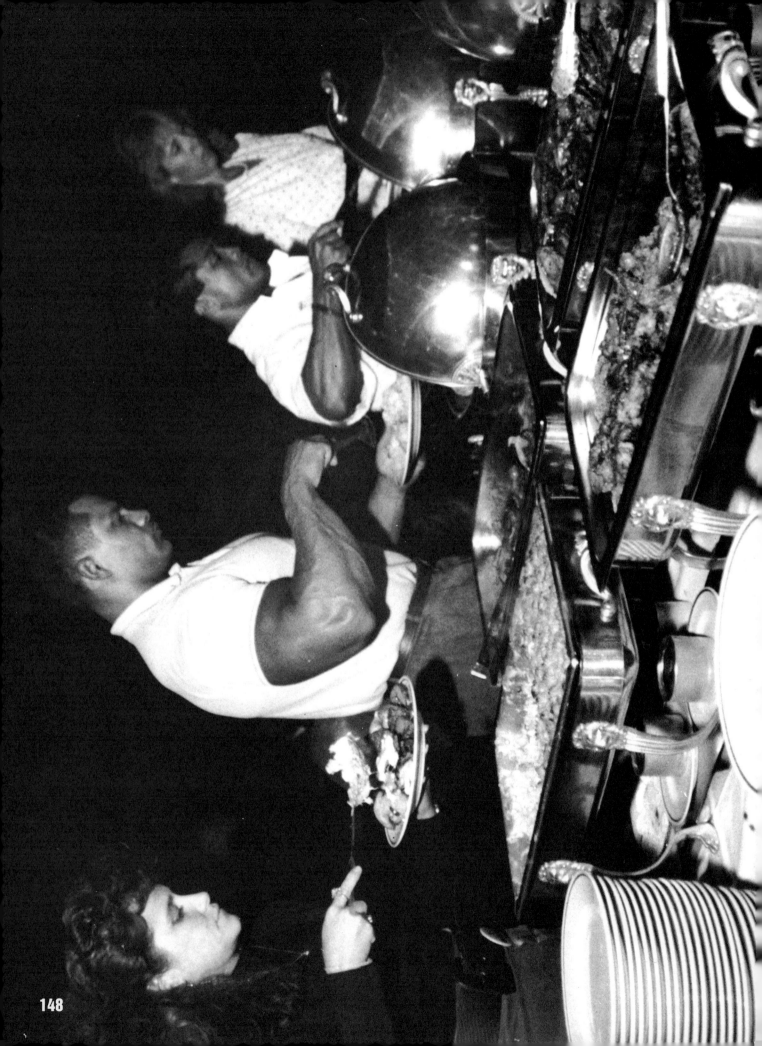

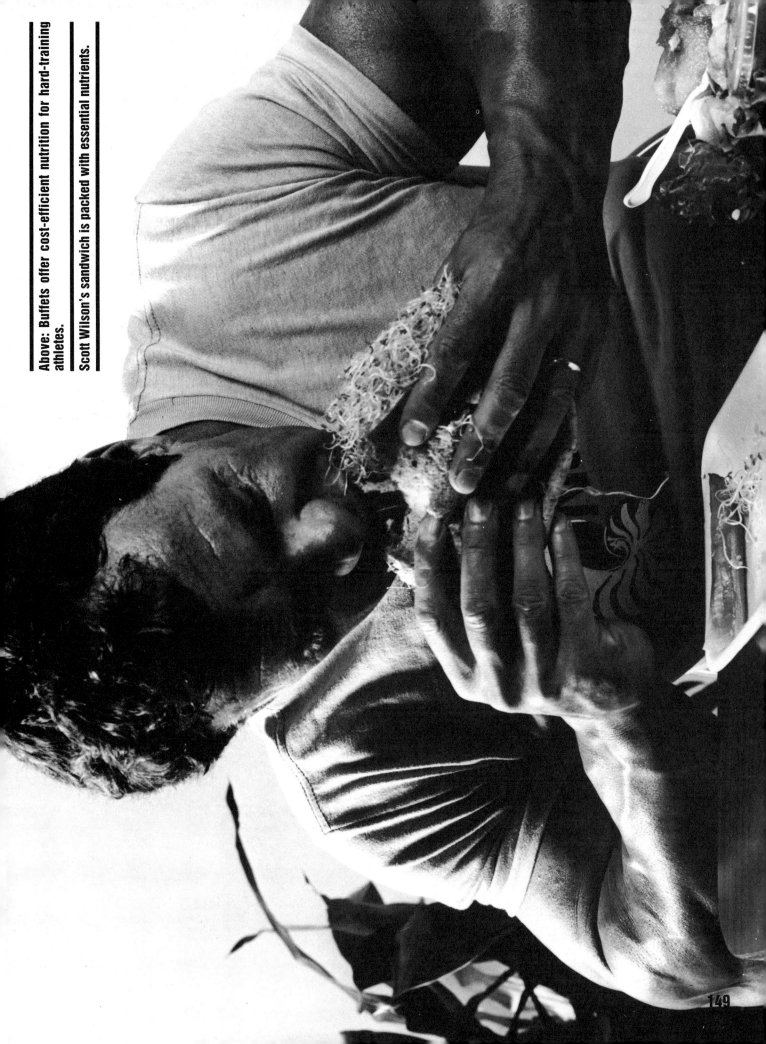

Above: Buffets offer cost-efficient nutrition for hard-training athletes.

Scott Wilson's sandwich is packed with essential nutrients.

Some bodybuilders each day consume dozens of nutrient pills, many of which have no positive effect on building muscle.

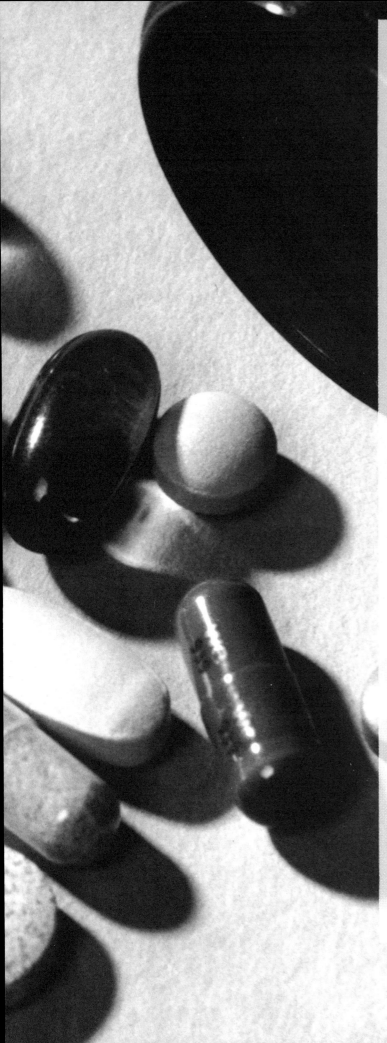

35 •
SUPPLEMENTS

If you read the muscle magazines, then you know that food supplements are big business. Statistics show that the sales of food supplements generate 30 times as much money as do the sales of exercise equipment. Look at the advertising in the various muscle magazines—you'll notice that a disproportionally large amount of space is devoted to food supplements.

Why are supplements such big business? Generally, it has to do with repeat sales. How many times can you sell a guy a 300-pound barbell set? Only once, because it doesn't wear out. But how many times can you sell him a bottle of vitamin pills or a can of amino acid tablets? Many times, if you can get him hooked.

In 1972 I reviewed all the published research on food supplements and bodybuilding for a postdoctoral nutrition study. I could not find a single study that convinced me that food supplements could build muscles any bigger or faster than common foods in a well-balanced eating plan.

Now it's some 20 years later and thousands of new supplements have been introduced—including such exotic names as chromium picolinate, vanadyl sulfate, and yohimbe bark—and I still find no scientific studies to convince me of the muscle-building powers of supplements.

Yes, there is research to show that antioxidants in concentrated form—such as vitamins C and E and beta-carotene—can possibly prevent certain diseases and improve longevity. Maybe you should investigate antioxidants if you're interested in living longer.

But if you're interested in building muscle, then supplements are not part of the answer.

You're much better off saving your money. What you can do is learn to read nutrition labels accurately so you can select your supermarket foods more intelligently.

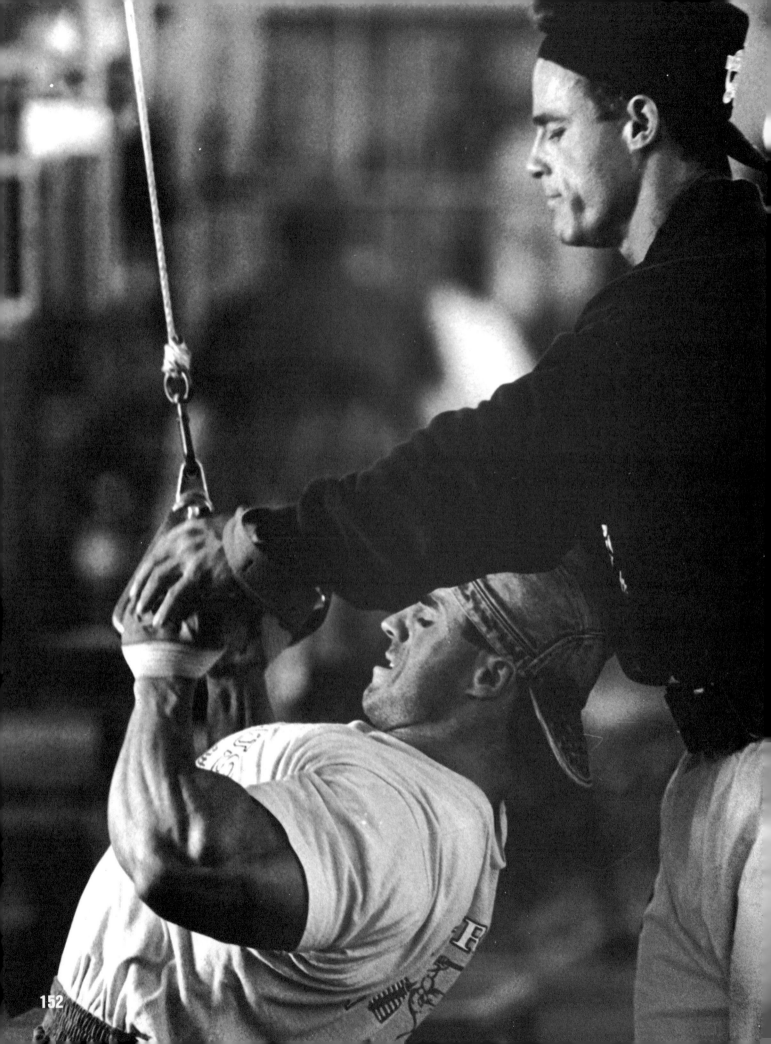

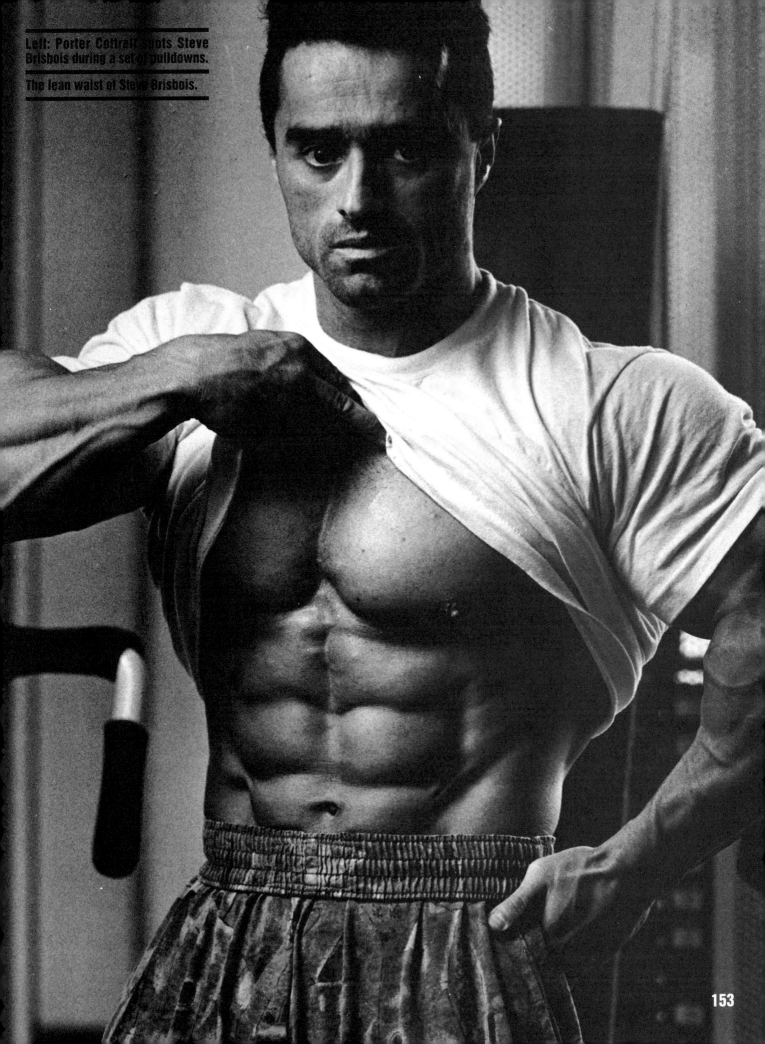

Left: Porter Cottrell shots Steve Brisbois during a set of pulldowns.

The lean waist of Steve Brisbois.

36 • STEROIDS

"Between two to three million Americans are currently using anabolic steroids," according to Bill Phillips, editor of Muscle Media 2000 magazine. "And it's a safe bet that for every one person who is using anabolic steroids, there's two or three who would like to be using them if they could get their hands on the drug. The demands for anabolic steroids far exceed their supply."

Steroid abuse is rampant in almost all sports where strength, speed, or size is important. Despite a long list of potential life-threatening risks, altered psychological behaviors, and much negative publicity associated with steroids, the demand is still prevalent. But why?

Mark Asanovich, a high school strength coach from Minnesota writing in the HIT Newsletter, says that our society promotes such abuse. He notes that society, in general, is drug oriented, performance oriented, appearance oriented, and now oriented. Is it any wonder that many young men fall into the getting-bigger-with-steroids mind-set?

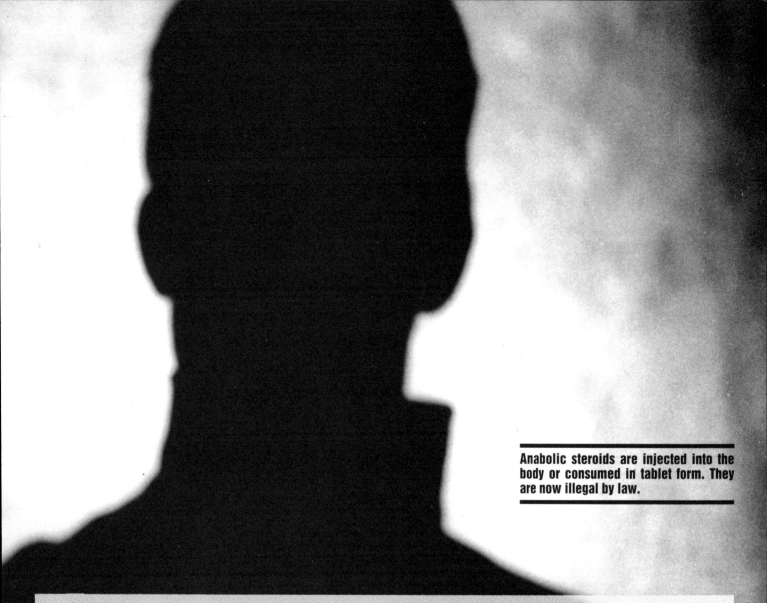

Anabolic steroids are injected into the body or consumed in tablet form. They are now illegal by law.

The situation was so bad that in 1990 the government stepped into the picture. According to the Federal Anabolic Steroid Control Act, it is a felony not only to use or possess steroids but to encourage someone to do so. For the most part, it is now illegal for physicians to prescribe steroids.

This government ban did much to boost the black market steroid industry, which mostly is made up of counterfeit drugs. Bill Phillips estimates that there are as many as 200 separate counterfeit suppliers in the United States alone. These counterfeiters procure a sample of the legitimate product and then have the label, box, and insert reprinted. As for what goes into these products, 90 percent contain no steroid ingredients at all. Most counterfeit versions of injectable steroids contain vegetable oil. Most tablets contain fillers such as potassium and calcium. Many are even packaged under unsanitary conditions.

The solution to this newest steroid problem and to all problems of steriod abuse are:

- Do not take or get involved with anabolic steroids. Most of those available through the black market—bodybuilding gyms and foreign mail-order—are counterfeit.
- Understand that anabolic steroids are potentially dangerous, life-threatening drugs.
- Realize that it is a felony to possess, use, or encourage the use of anabolic steroids. In other words, it is against the law!
- Rise above the clouded priorities of our drug-, performance-, appearance-, and now-oriented society.
- Learn to believe in the basics of high-intensity exercise, well-balanced nutrition, and adequate rest. Your subsequent muscle growth will surprise you!

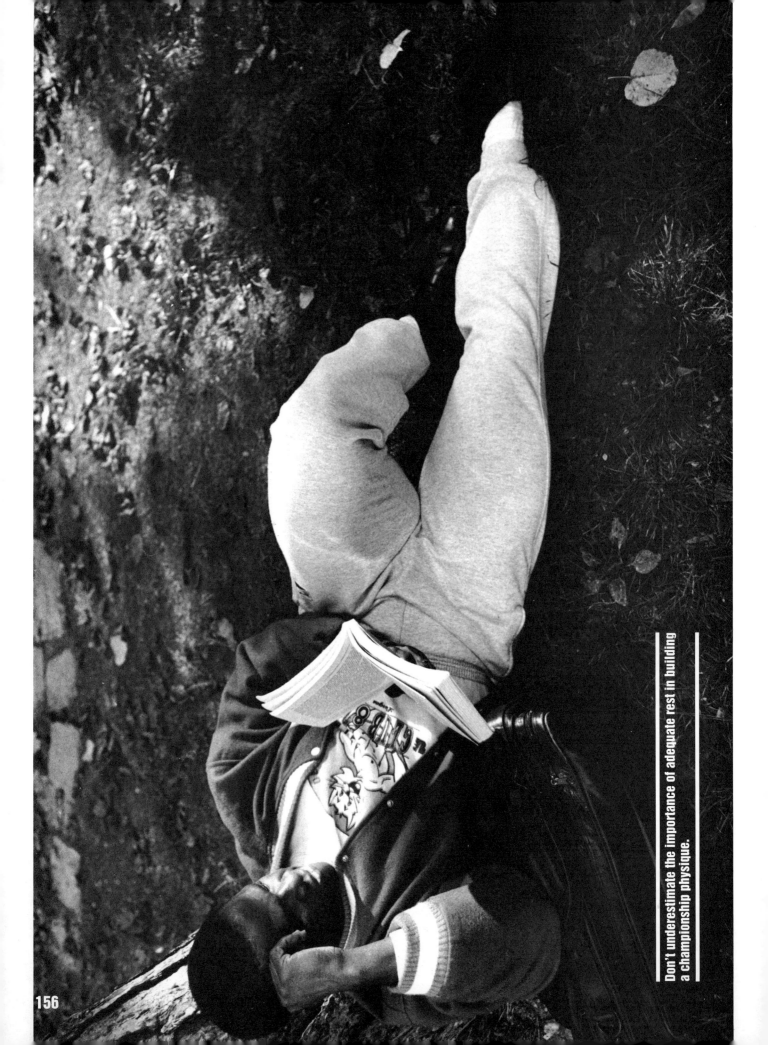

Don't underestimate the importance of adequate rest in building a championship physique.

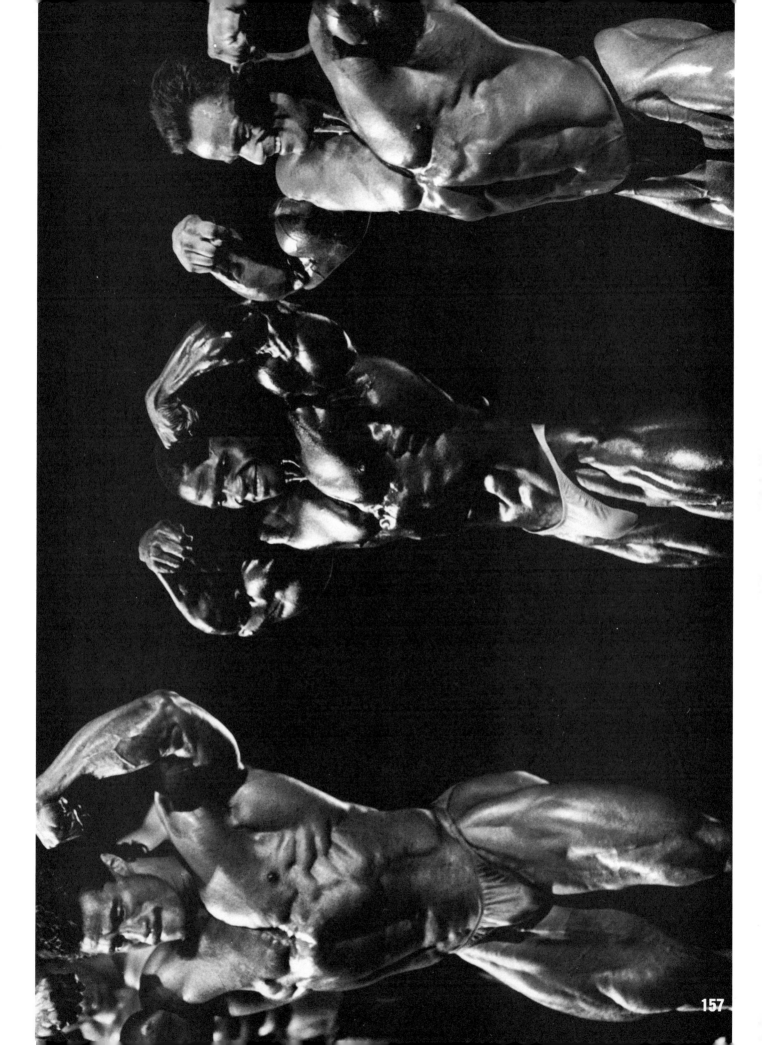

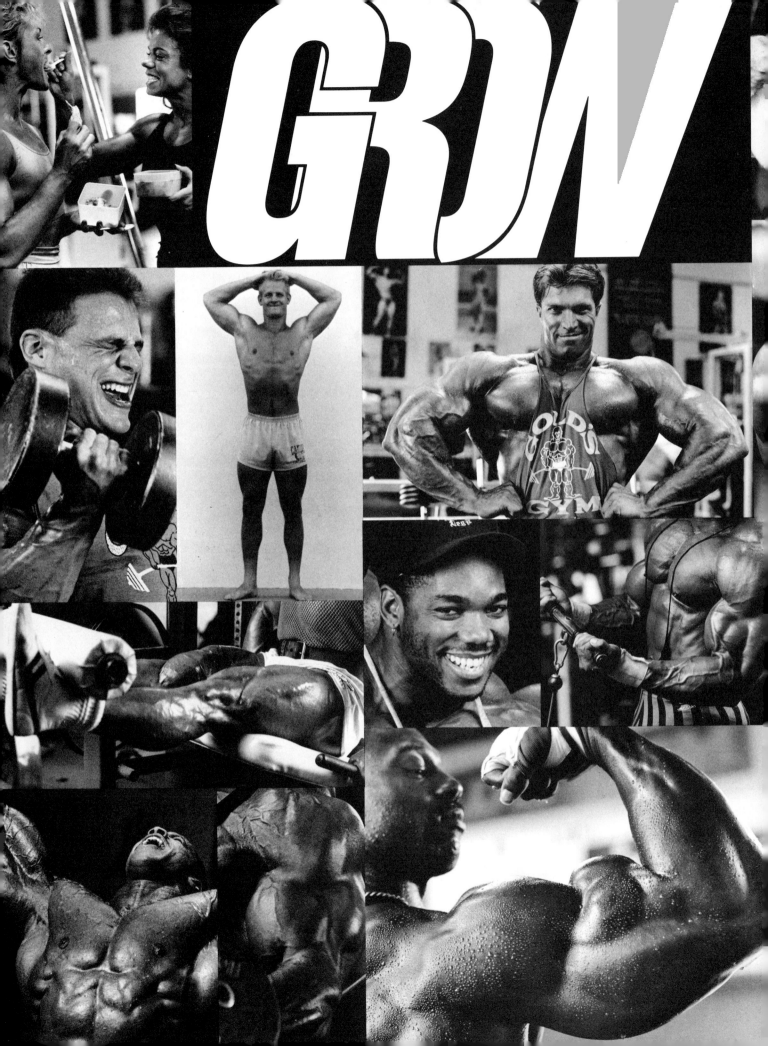

GROW

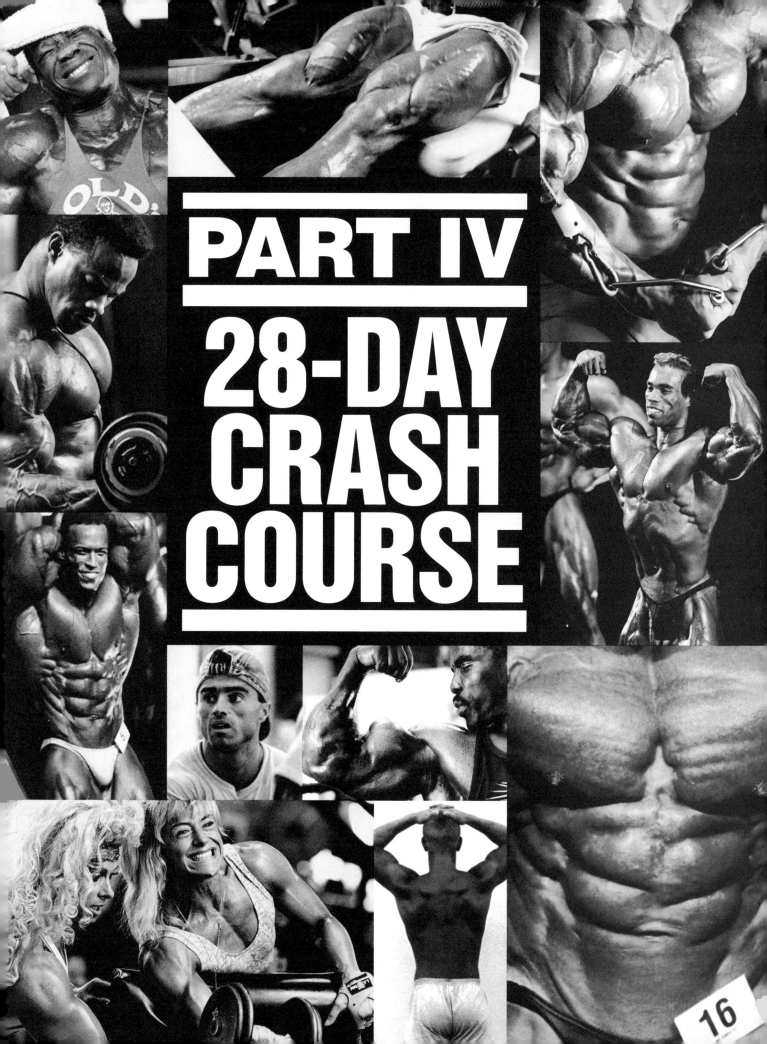

PART IV

28-DAY CRASH COURSE

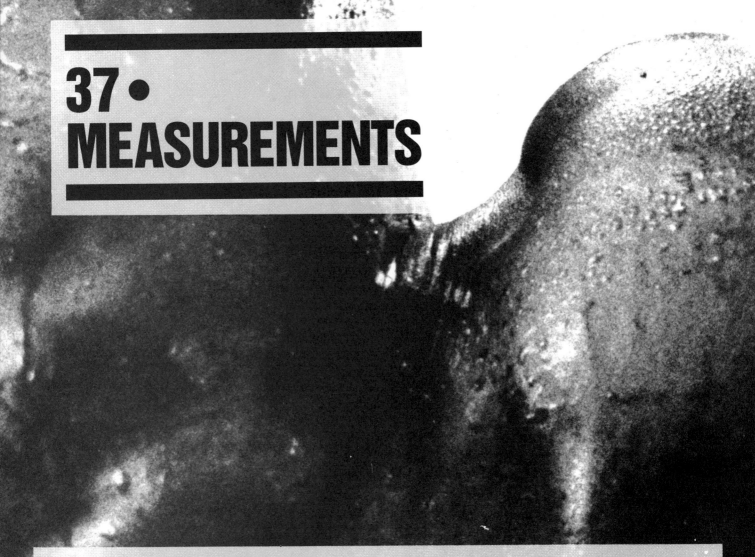

37 • MEASUREMENTS

Many athletes and bodybuilders train at the Gainesville Health & Fitness Center in Gainesville, Florida. In May of 1992 I recruited Jeff Turner, a 19-year-old athlete who used the facility and who also played football for the University of Florida. I knew from observing Jeff in some of his exercises that he was a hard worker. Plus, he wanted to put on as much muscle as he could for the approaching football season.

The next seven chapters detail how I measured, organized, trained, and evaluated Jeff Turner through a 28-day muscle-building crash course. I integrated all the principles from Parts I, II, and III into the program.

Before getting started it is important to take the following measurements: height, weight, circumferences at 12 sites, and percent body fat.

For your circumferences, get a 60-inch plastic tape and a pencil, read through the following directions, and record the numbers on page 162. Apply the tape firmly to the skin but do not compress it. You'll get more accurate numbers if your training partner does the measurements for you.

Neck: Circle the tape around the neck at the level just above the Adam's apple.

Upper arms: Bend the elbow and contract the right biceps with the upper arm parallel to the floor. Pass the tape around the largest part of the contracted biceps. Do the same for the left arm.

Forearms: With the right elbow straight, make a fist, bend the wrist, and contract the forearm. Do the same for the left forearm.

Chest: Stretch the tape around the back at nipple level and bring it together in front. Breathe normally and take the reading.

Waist: Loop the tape around the waist at navel level. Do not pull in the belly.

Hips: Circle the tape around the hips at the level of maximum protrusion of the buttocks. Keep the feet together.

Thighs: Place the feet shoulder-width apart. Pass the tape around the right thigh just below the buttocks. Keep the thigh relaxed. Do the same for the left thigh.

Calves: Place the feet shoulder-width apart. Circle the tape around the right calf at the largest

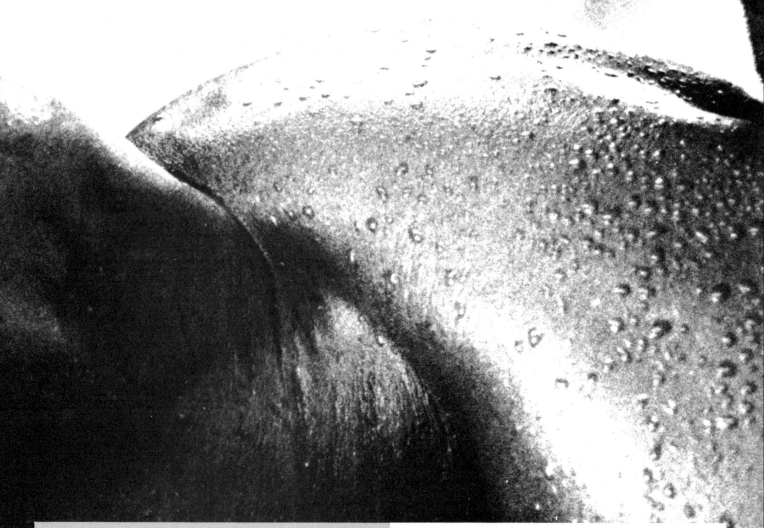

point. Keep the muscle relaxed. Do the same for the left calf.

For determining your percent body fat, use a Lange skinfold caliper (if available) to measure the thickness of your skin and fat at three positions: men — chest, navel, and thigh; women — triceps, hip, and thigh. A special nomogram from <u>Research Quarterly for Exercise and Sport</u> 52: 380–384, (1981) may be applied to the sum to determine the percentage of body fat. You should be able to locate this journal at a research library.

Full-body photographs are another important way to judge progress. Have photographs taken of yourself in brief trunks. Stand against an uncluttered background with your hands on your head and your feet apart evenly. You'll be surprised by what will happen throughout your body in your front and back poses after only 28 days.

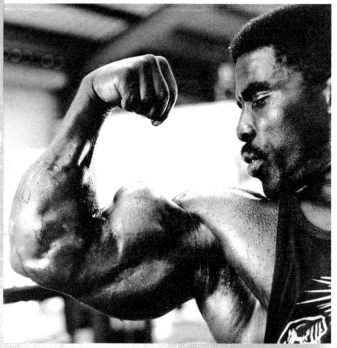

No one in bodybuilding has a higher peaked biceps than Robby Robinson.

GROW: THE 28-DAY MUSCLE-BUILDING CRASH COURSE

NAME _____ AGE _____

	BEFORE	AFTER	DIFFERENCE
Date	_____	_____	
Height	_____	_____	
Weight	_____	_____	_____
Circumference Measurements	_____	_____	_____
Neck	_____	_____	_____
Right upper arm	_____	_____	_____
Left upper arm	_____	_____	_____
Right forearm	_____	_____	_____
Left forearm	_____	_____	_____
Chest	_____	_____	_____
Waist	_____	_____	_____
Hips	_____	_____	_____
Right thigh	_____	_____	_____
Left thigh	_____	_____	_____
Right calf	_____	_____	_____
Left calf	_____	_____	_____
Skinfold Measurements	_____	_____	_____
Right chest	_____	_____	_____
Right abdomen	_____	_____	_____
Right thigh	_____	_____	_____
Total	_____	_____	_____
Percentage	_____	_____	_____

Photographs: front, side, back

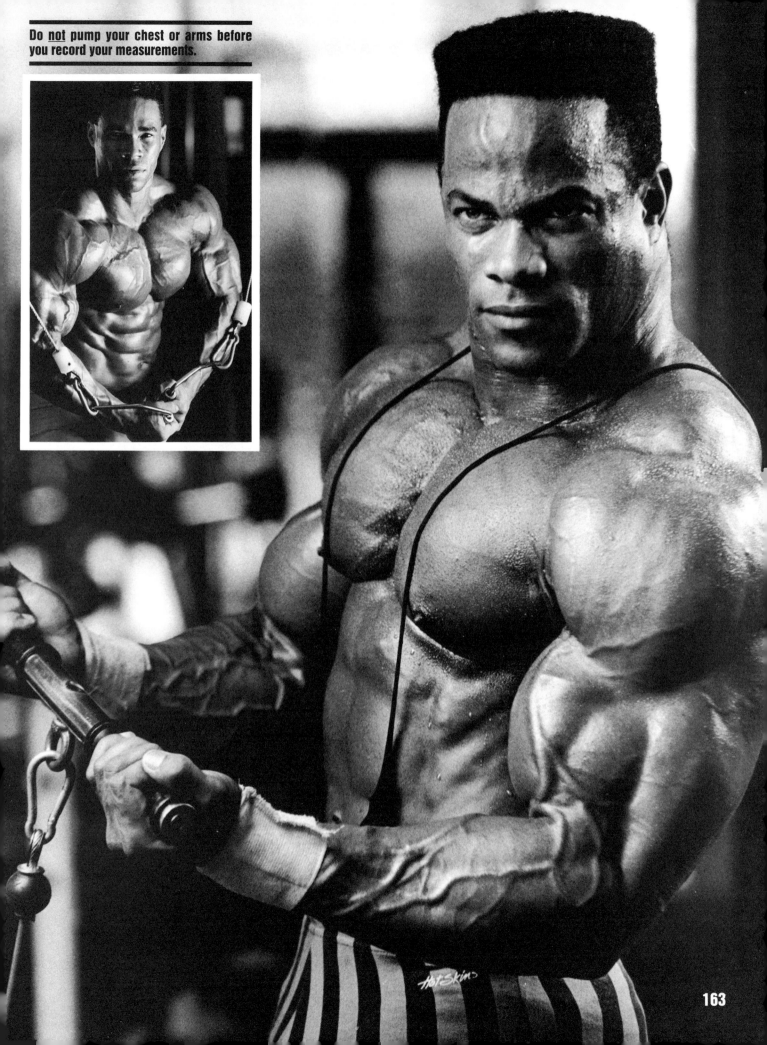

Do not pump your chest or arms before you record your measurements.

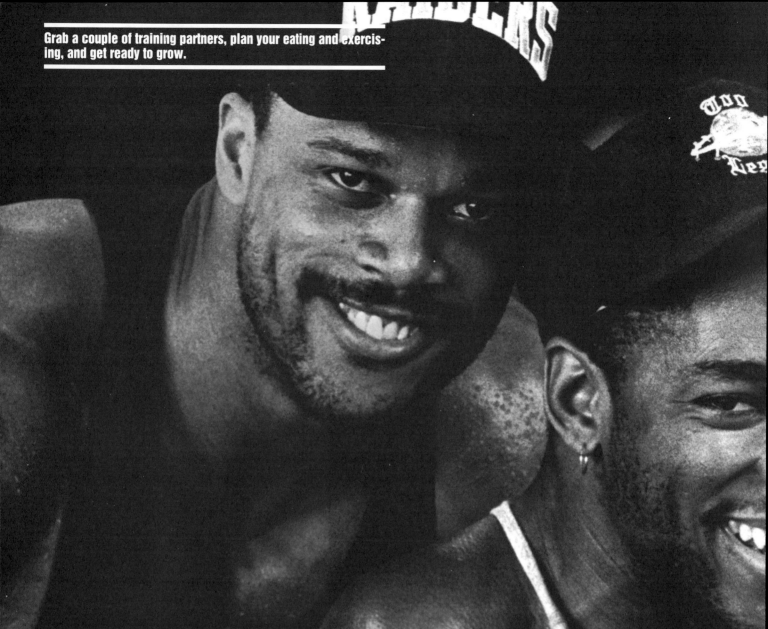

Grab a couple of training partners, plan your eating and exercising, and get ready to grow.

38 •
THE COURSE

The 28-day exercising and eating course is divided into four one-week segments. The Week One exercise plan consists of a basic, whole-body routine. Week Two concentrates on the lower body. Week Three emphasizes the back and chest, and Week Four focuses on the arms.

The four-week eating plan is a bit more complex. I took Jeff Turner to Dr. Robert Cade's laboratory at the University of Florida College of Medicine to determine his resting metabolic rate. At a height of 6 feet and a weight of 186.7 pounds, Jeff burned 2,367 calories a day in a relaxed state.

To estimate the number of calories that Jeff would require for maximum growth, I had to account for his work activity, exercise intensity and duration, and digestion efficiency. Jeff was involved in light construction work so I added 60 percent of his resting rate, or 1,420 calories. I figured his workouts at 300 calories each and his digestion at another 300. The total came to 4,387 calories, which seemed a little high. Since in my last several bodybuilding projects I've overestimated the calories slightly, I decided to lower Jeff's somewhat. I wanted to be sure that he put on a minimum amount of fat in the growth process.

Thus, I decided that Jeff's daily calorie consumption should be:

4,300 calories for Week One
4,400 calories for Week Two
4,500 calories for Week Three
4,600 calories for Week Four

As I mentioned previously, Stacey Goss of Computerized Bodyweight Management Systems was very helpful in planning Jeff's day-to-day menus. She had Jeff examine a master list and indicate the foods that he liked to eat. For example, there were 38 choices under the <u>fruit</u> section and 49 selections under <u>cold cereals</u>.

Once Jeff made his choices in all the categories, everything was entered into a computer that had been programmed with the chemical composition of the listed foods and products. Stacey instructed the computer to provide daily menus using Jeff's selections with a breakdown of 60 percent carbohydrates, 15 percent proteins, and 25 percent fats. A one-day example for each week is shown in the next four chapters.

Included in Jeff's dietary schedule was an in-between-meal snack called Go! Quick-Shake. Go! was invented by Dr. Robert Cade, the man behind Gatorade. It is available in an eight-ounce, shelf-stable carton and contains 190 calories. Go! is manufactured by Phoenix Advanced Technology and it is distributed by Marketshare International. For information, call (800) 972-2020.

If you'd like Stacey Goss's help in organizing a nutritious eating plan, please write to Computerized Bodyweight Management Systems, P.O. Box 62597, Colorado Springs, CO 80962, or call (800) 743-9750, for further information.

What can you do if you don't have access to equipment that measures your metabolic rate, and if you don't have time to get computerized menus for yourself?

For estimating daily calorie expenditure, I've used a simple formula for over 20 years that works well: multiply your body weight in pounds by 20. If you weigh 160 pounds, for example, then 160×20 equals 3,200 calories per day to maintain your body weight.

To grow—to build muscle—however, you need extra calories. How much more? Here are the guidelines according to your body weight:

- 175 pounds or under, add 400 calories
- 176–200 pounds, add 500 calories
- 201 pounds or over, add 600 calories

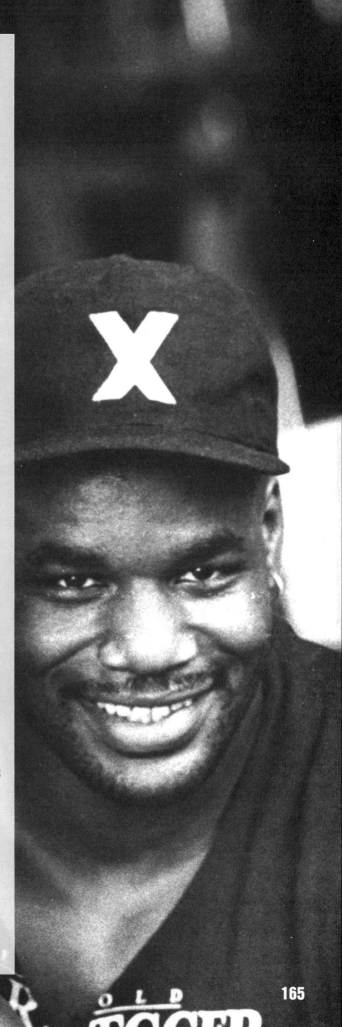

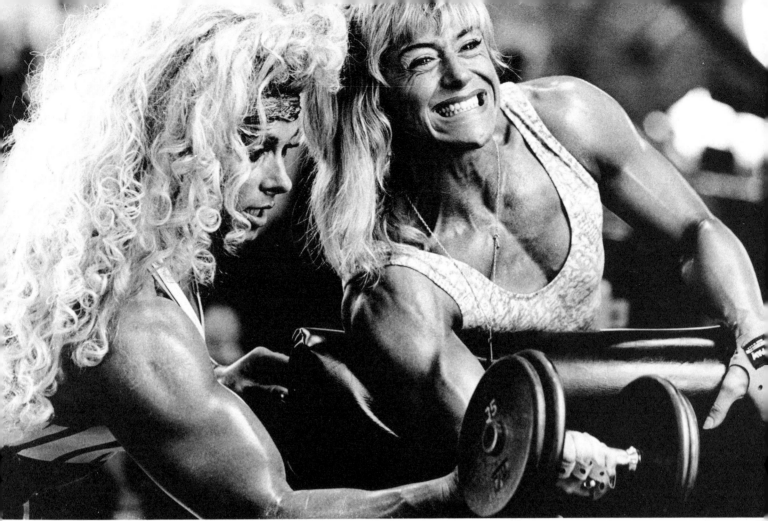

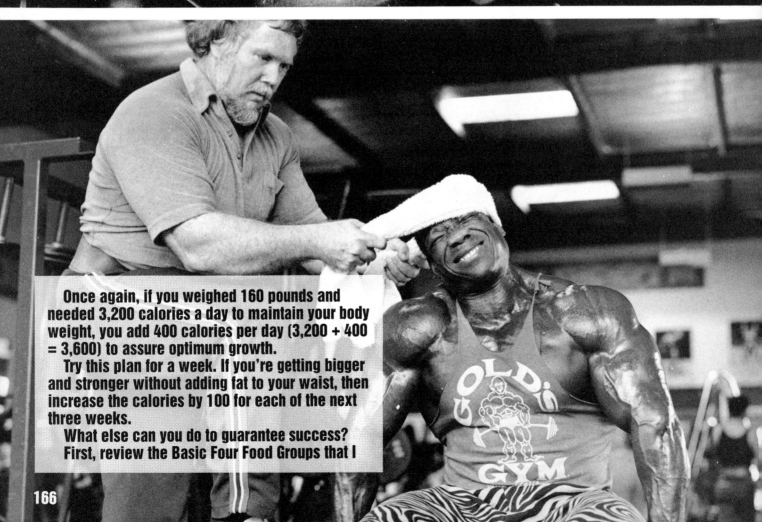

Once again, if you weighed 160 pounds and needed 3,200 calories a day to maintain your body weight, you add 400 calories per day (3,200 + 400 = 3,600) to assure optimum growth.

Try this plan for a week. If you're getting bigger and stronger without adding fat to your waist, then increase the calories by 100 for each of the next three weeks.

What else can you do to guarantee success?

First, review the Basic Four Food Groups that I

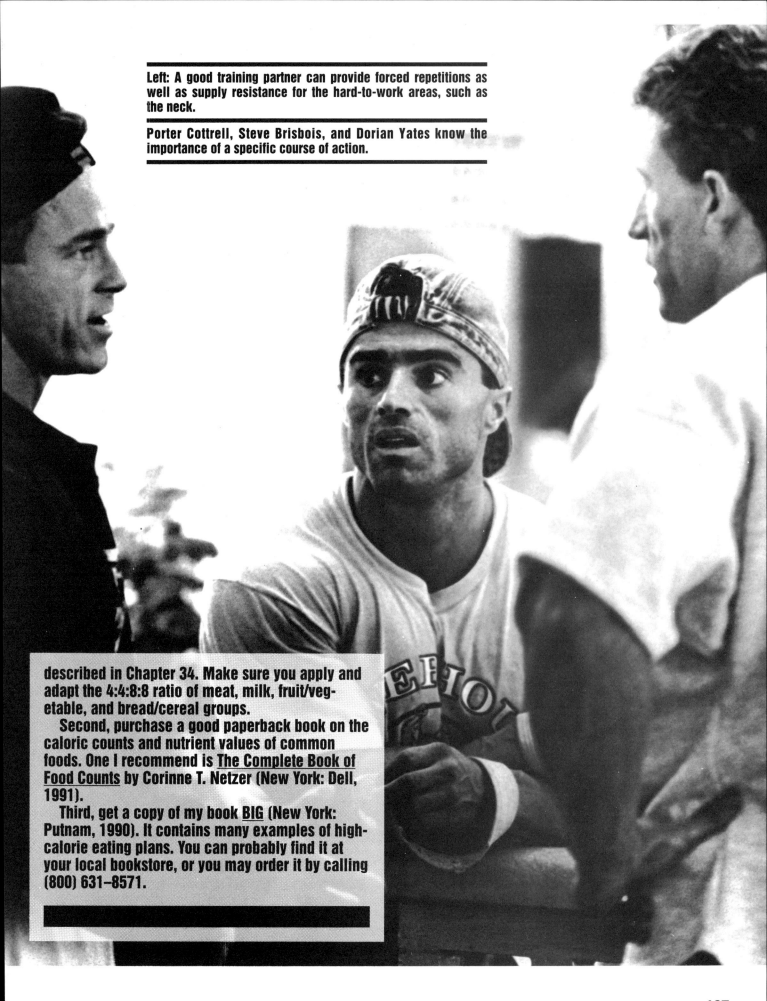

Left: A good training partner can provide forced repetitions as well as supply resistance for the hard-to-work areas, such as the neck.

Porter Cottrell, Steve Brisbois, and Dorian Yates know the importance of a specific course of action.

described in Chapter 34. Make sure you apply and adapt the 4:4:8:8 ratio of meat, milk, fruit/vegetable, and bread/cereal groups.

Second, purchase a good paperback book on the caloric counts and nutrient values of common foods. One I recommend is <u>The Complete Book of Food Counts</u> by Corinne T. Netzer (New York: Dell, 1991).

Third, get a copy of my book <u>BIG</u> (New York: Putnam, 1990). It contains many examples of high-calorie eating plans. You can probably find it at your local bookstore, or you may order it by calling (800) 631–8571.

For the next four weeks, you'll be exercising on a Monday-Wednesday-Friday schedule. It is important that you rest and recover as much as is reasonably possible on Tuesday, Thursday, Saturday, and Sunday. Remember, your muscles grow on your nontraining days.

Week One consists of a basic, total body routine. You can return to this routine again and again as it is simple and produces results. Here's a brief exercise-by-exercise description of your basic workout.

1. <u>Leg curl machine</u>. Lie face down on the leg curl machine and place your heels under the roller pads. Bend your knees and try to touch your heels to your buttocks. Pause. Lower smoothly to the stretched position. Repeat for maximum repetitions.

2. <u>Leg extension machine</u>. Straighten your legs smoothly to full extension. Pause. Lower and repeat until you reach momentary muscle fatigue.

3. <u>Squat with barbell</u>. With a barbell behind your neck and across your shoulders, bend your hips and knees and lower your buttocks until the backs of your thighs touch your calves. Return smoothly to the top and repeat.

4. <u>Standing calf raise machine</u>. Raise your heels smoothly and stand on your tiptoes. Pause. Lower for a stretch. Repeat until fatigued.

5. <u>Overhead press with barbell</u>. Press the barbell smoothly in front of your face and over your head. Lower slowly and repeat.

6. <u>Pullover on machine</u>. Use a Nautilus pullover machine if you have one or a bent-armed pullover with a barbell if you don't. Do as many repetitions as you can.

7. <u>Dip</u>. On the parallel bars, do as many smooth dips as possible.

8. <u>Bent-over row with barbell</u>. Pull the barbell upward until it touches your lower ribs. Return for a stretch and repeat.

9. <u>Triceps extension with one dumbbell</u>. Hold a dumbbell at one end with both hands and press it overhead. Lower the dumbbell slowly behind your neck. Straighten your elbows smoothly and repeat.

10. <u>Biceps curl with barbell</u>. Curl a heavy barbell strictly as many repetitions as possible.

11. <u>Bent-kneed sit-up</u>. With your knees bent, hook your feet at the top of a sit-up board. Do slow, smooth sit-ups until you're fatigued.

12. <u>4-way neck machine</u>. Use a Nautilus or Hammer neck machine for this exercise. Work only the back and front sections of your neck.

13. <u>Shoulder shrug with barbell</u>. With a heavy barbell in your hands, shrug your shoulders as high as possible. Repeat.

The following workout chart has boxes to the right of the exercises to record your resistance and repetitions for the three weekly training sessions.

GROW: 28-DAY CRASH COURSE DAYS 1-7: BASIC OVERALL BODY ROUTINE			
Exercise	Date Body Weight		
1. Leg curl			
2. Leg extension			
3. Squat			
4. Calf raise			
5. Overhead press			
6. Pullover			
7. Dip			
8. Bent-over row			
9. Triceps extension			
10. Biceps curl			
11. Bent-kneed sit-up			
12. 4-way neck			
13. Shoulder shrug			
Name:			

The following menu sheet is an example of the 4,300-calorie-a-day eating plan that Jeff Turner utilized for Days 1–7. Your eating schedule should be similar.

Kevin Levrone, runner-up in the 1992 Mr. Olympia contest, and Dorian Yates, the winner.

DAILY MENU SHEET

NAME: Jeff Turner   **MONDAY**   **WEEK 1**

BREAKFAST	AMOUNT	CALORIES
Corn grits, instant, flavored	2 packets	205
Skim milk	1 cup	84
Strawberries, raw	2 cups	102
Bagel, any flavor	2	380
Margarine	5 teaspoons	171
Apple juice	12 ounces	178

MIDMORNING SNACK		
Angel food cake	1 piece	134
GO! Nutrition Quick-Shake	8 ounces	191

LUNCH		
Sandwich bread (any type)	4 slices	284
Tuna, water packed	2 ounces	69
Lettuce and tomato	unlimited	25
Mustard or low-calorie mayonnaise	6 teaspoons	99
Kiwi fruit, raw	3 medium	153
Graham crackers	2 ounces	228
Skim milk	1 cup	84

AFTERNOON SNACK		
Kiwi fruit, raw	2 medium	102
Cheddar cheese, reduced fat	1 ounce	81
GO! Nutrition Quick-Shake	8 ounces	191

DINNER		
Snapper, broiled or baked	2 ounces	69
Brown rice, cooked	1 cup	218
Margarine	6 teaspoons	205
Greens (any type), cooked	1 cup	40
Bread sticks	6	226
Margarine	6 teaspoons	205
Passion fruit juice	10 ounces	176

AFTER-DINNER SNACK		
Sandwich bread (any type)	2 slices	142
Peanut butter	1 tablespoon	81
Jelly or jam	6 teaspoons	96
Skim milk	1 cup	84

TOTAL CALORIES = 4,303

CARBOHYDRATES	649.2 grams	**PROTEIN**	168.9 grams	**FAT**	114.8 grams
% CARBOHYDRATES	60.3	**% PROTEIN**	15.7	**% FAT**	24.0

Some form of biceps curl should be a part of your total body routine.

Below: Dorian Yates and Shawn Ray compare their abdominals.

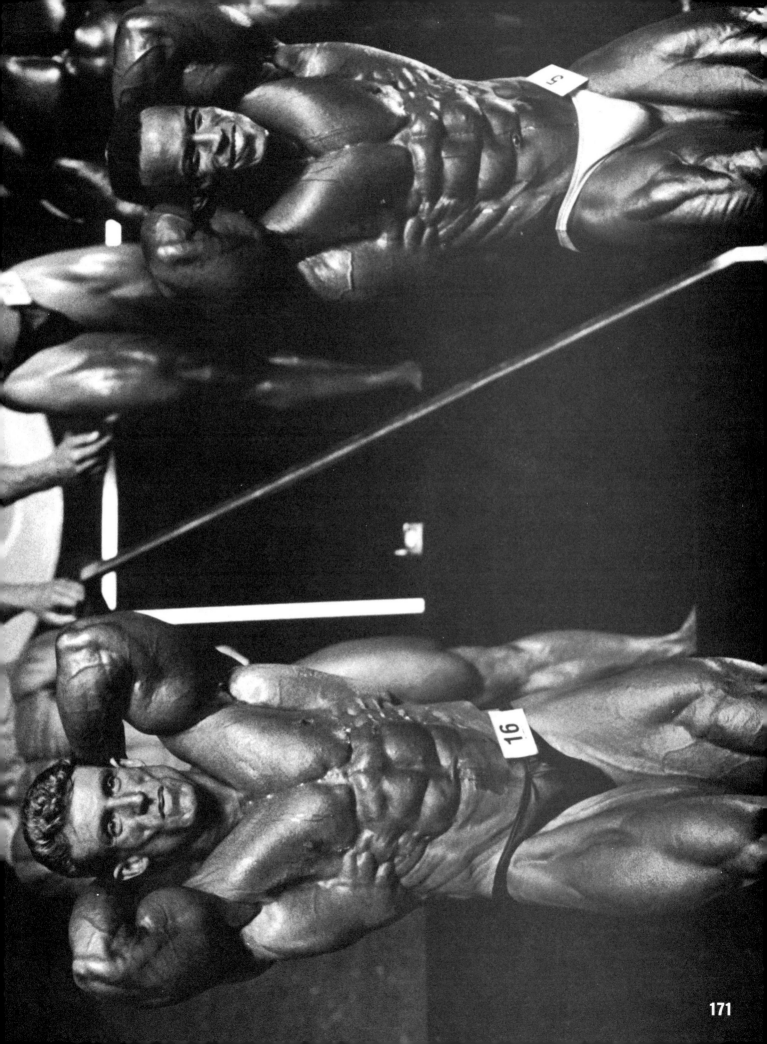

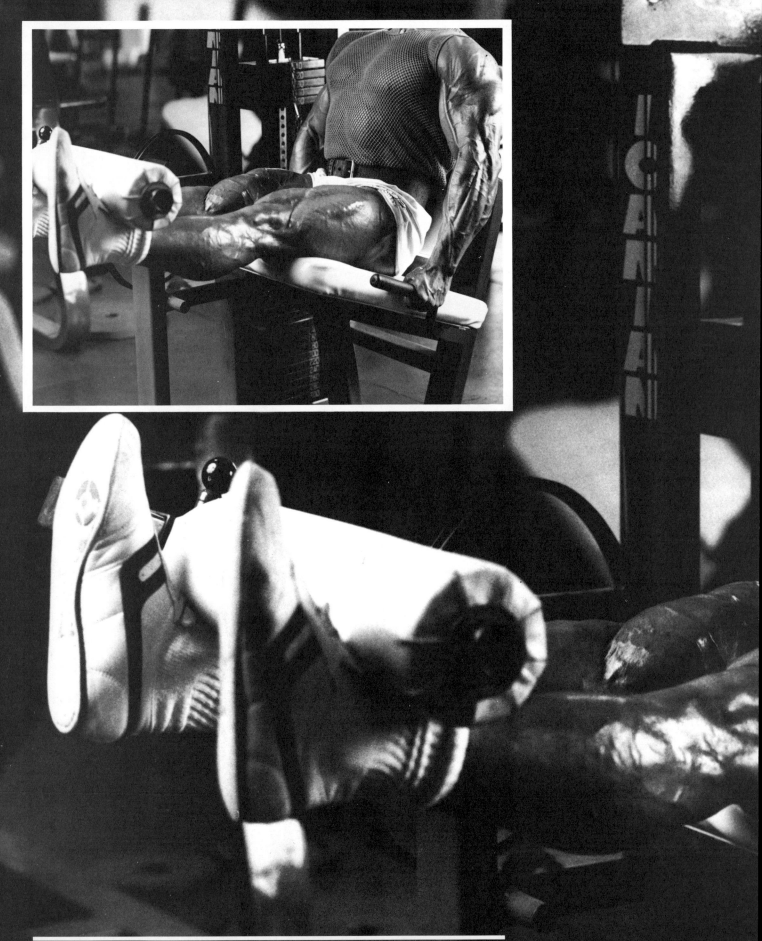

The leg extension provides approximately 120 degrees of rotary resistance around the knee joints. Always do each repetition slowly and smoothly.

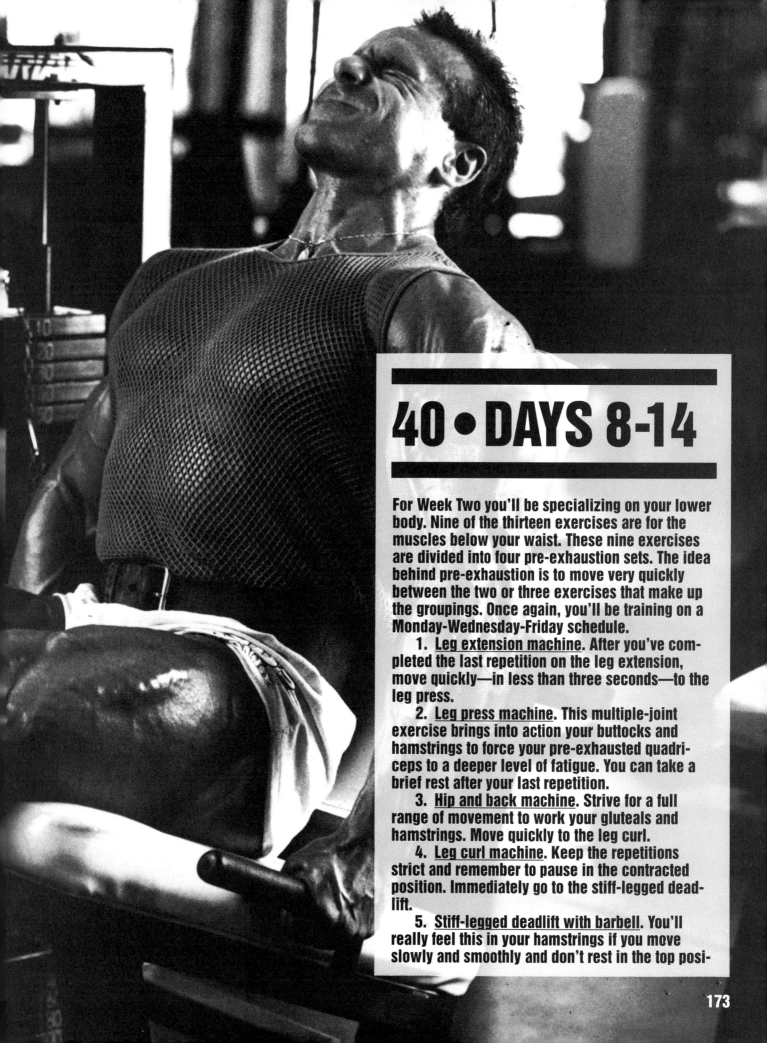

40 • DAYS 8-14

For Week Two you'll be specializing on your lower body. Nine of the thirteen exercises are for the muscles below your waist. These nine exercises are divided into four pre-exhaustion sets. The idea behind pre-exhaustion is to move very quickly between the two or three exercises that make up the groupings. Once again, you'll be training on a Monday-Wednesday-Friday schedule.

1. <u>Leg extension machine</u>. After you've completed the last repetition on the leg extension, move quickly—in less than three seconds—to the leg press.

2. <u>Leg press machine</u>. This multiple-joint exercise brings into action your buttocks and hamstrings to force your pre-exhausted quadriceps to a deeper level of fatigue. You can take a brief rest after your last repetition.

3. <u>Hip and back machine</u>. Strive for a full range of movement to work your gluteals and hamstrings. Move quickly to the leg curl.

4. <u>Leg curl machine</u>. Keep the repetitions strict and remember to pause in the contracted position. Immediately go to the stiff-legged deadlift.

5. <u>Stiff-legged deadlift with barbell</u>. You'll really feel this in your hamstrings if you move slowly and smoothly and don't rest in the top posi-

tion. Grind out as many repetitions as possible and take another brief rest.

6. <u>Standing calf raise machine.</u> Do the standing and seated calf raise back to back. Keep your knees locked on the standing calf raise.

7. <u>Seated calf raise machine.</u> With your knees bent, raise and lower your heels until momentary muscle fatigue. Rest your calves briefly.

8. <u>Hip abduction machine.</u> You'll feel this machine working the outsides of your buttocks.

9. <u>Hip adduction machines.</u> Concentrate on pulling with your knees and thighs, not your ankles.

10. <u>Lateral raise with dumbbells.</u> Raise the dumbbells to shoulder height at your sides. Pause. Lower slowly and repeat.

11. <u>Pullover on machine.</u> Again, do the pullover with a Nautilus machine or a barbell.

12. <u>Bench press with barbell.</u> Keep all your repetitions slow and smooth.

13. <u>Biceps curl with barbell:</u> Give this final exercise your best effort.

GROW: 28-DAY CRASH COURSE DAYS 8–14: LOWER-BODY SPECIALIZATION				
Exercise	Date Body Weight			
1. Leg extension				
2. Leg press				
3. Hip and back				
4. Leg curl				
5. Stiff-legged deadlift				
6. Calf raise				
7. Seated calf raise				
8. Hip abduction				
9. Hip adduction				
10. Lateral raise				
11. Pullover				
12. Bench press				
13. Biceps curl				
Name:				

Note: Perform the exercises inside the brackets with no rest in between.

To support the lower body specialization routine, Jeff's daily eating plan was increased by 100 calories per day. He consumed 4,400 calories during days 8–14. The following is an example of his typical menu breakdown:

The quadriceps, as the name implies, is composed of four large muscles.

DAILY MENU SHEET

NAME: Jeff Turner | **SUNDAY** | **WEEK 2**

BREAKFAST

	AMOUNT	CALORIES
Homemade pancakes, plain	8	492
Margarine	6 teaspoons	205
Syrup	3 ounces	312
Strawberries, raw	1.5 cups	77
Skim milk	1 cup	84
Passion fruit juice	12 ounces	211

MIDMORNING SNACK

Rye bread	2 slices	146
Jelly or jam	2 teaspoons	32
GO! Nutrition Quick-Shake	8 ounces	191

LUNCH

Tomato soup	2.5 cups	223
Bread sticks	6	226
Margarine	2 teaspoons	68
Cheddar cheese, reduced fat	2 ounces	162
Plum, raw	3 medium	120

AFTERNOON SNACK

Instant pudding, sugar-free	1 cup	206
GO! Nutrition Quick-Shake	8 ounces	191
GO! Nutrition Quick-Shake	8 ounces	191

DINNER

Lasagna	12 ounces	563
Tossed salad (raw vegetables only)	1 large	74
Low-calorie salad dressing	3 tablespoons	105
Apple juice	10 ounces	149

AFTER-DINNER SNACK

Raisin bran cereal	3 ounces	304
Skim milk	1 cup	84

TOTAL CALORIES = 4,416

CARBOHYDRATES	673.1 grams	**PROTEIN**	168.5 grams	**FAT**	117.2 grams
% CARBOHYDRATES	61.0	**% PROTEIN**	15.2	**% FAT**	23.9

At the start of day 15 of the program, Jeff's body weight had gone from 186.7 to 198.5 pounds. That was an increase of 11.8 pounds in 14 days.

Your body weight also should be increasing. You most definitely should be growing.

During days 15–21 you'll specialize on your back and chest. You'll be applying pre-exhaustion sets on both these large body parts. Here's your Monday-Wednesday-Friday exercise routine:

1. **Bent-over row with barbell.** The first two pre-exhaustion cycles involve doing three exercises each, back to back, with no rest in between. Be sure to arrange your equipment accordingly. Do the bent-over row until exhaustion. Move quickly to the pullover.

2. **Negative pullover.** Load up a heavier-than-normal weight on the Nautilus pullover. Get your training partner to assist you to the contracted position. Lower the resistance slowly in 10 seconds to the stretched position. Repeat for at least 8 repetitions. Get to the pulldown immediately.

3. **Pulldown on lat machine.** Use a narrow underhanded grip and pull the bar to your chest. Lower slowly and repeat until you reach muscle fatigue. Take a brief rest and ready yourself for the chest cycle.

4. **Incline press with barbell.** On an incline bench, lift and lower the barbell to your upper chest. After the last repetition, move to the bent-armed fly.

5. **Bent-armed fly with dumbbells.** Perform the flying movement slowly and smoothly. Now do the push-up.

6. **Push-up.** Quickly assume a prone position on the floor with your hands under your shoulders. Do as many slow push-ups as possible. If you can complete more than 10, elevate your feet to increase the difficulty.

7. **Negative chin-up.** With an underhanded grip, climb into the top position of a chin-up. Remove your feet from the step and lower your body slowly in 10 seconds. Repeat.

8. **Negative dip.** Climb into the top position of a dip. Remove your feet from the step and lower your body slowly in 10 seconds. Repeat.

9. **Shoulder shrug with barbell.** Raise and lower your shoulders for maximum repetitions.

10. **4-way neck.** Do only the right and left sides of your neck for this week.

11. **Leg curl machine.** Your hamstrings should be growing stronger as a result of this isolation movement.

12. **Leg extension machine.** This single-joint exercise for your quadriceps will leave them exhausted.

13. **Hip adduction machine.** Your inner thighs will feel this unique movement.

GROW: 28-DAY CRASH COURSE
DAYS 15–21: BACK-CHEST SPECIALIZATION

Exercise Date / Body Weight			
1. Bent-over row			
2. Negative pullover			
3. Pulldown			
4. Incline press			
5. Bent-armed fly			
6. Push-up			
7. Negative chin-up			
8. Negative dip			
9. Shoulder shrug			
10. 4-way neck			
11. Leg curl			
12. Leg extension			
13. Hip adduction			
Name:			

Note: Perform the exercises inside the brackets with no rest in between.

According to plans, you should be adding an additional 100 calories per day to menus for Week Three. An example of one of Jeff's menus for days 15–21 is as follows.

Your chest and back are the targeted body parts for Week 3.

DAILY MENU SHEET

NAME: Jeff Turner | **SATURDAY** | **WEEK 3**

BREAKFAST	AMOUNT	CALORIES
Grape-Nuts cereal	2 ounces	216
Skim milk	1 cup	84
Pineapple, juice pack	1 cup	163
Raisin bread	2 slices	140
Margarine	5 teaspoons	171
Cranberry juice	10 ounces	174

MIDMORNING SNACK		
Watermelon, raw	2 cups	113
Lowfat yogurt, flavored	6 ounces	172
GO! Nutrition Quick-Shake	8 ounces	191

LUNCH		
Macaroni and cheese	2 cups	692
Sandwich bread (any type)	4 slices	284
Bacon, lean only	2 slices	71
Lettuce and tomato	unlimited	25
Mustard or low-calorie mayonnaise	6 teaspoons	99
Peach, raw	2 medium	84
Nabisco Cheese Nips	1 ounce	134

AFTERNOON SNACK		
Orange, raw	2 medium	136
GO! Nutrition Quick-Shake	8 ounces	191
GO! Nutrition Quick-Shake	8 ounces	191

DINNER		
Turkey, breast	2 ounces	102
Baked beans	1/2 cup	134
Green beans, cooked	2 cups	105
Kaiser roll	1	194
Margarine	6 teaspoons	205
Orange juice	8 ounces	108

AFTER-DINNER SNACK		
Microwave natural popcorn, light	3 cups	53
GO! Nutrition Quick-Shake	8 ounces	191
Skim milk	1 cup	84

TOTAL CALORIES = 4,507

CARBOHYDRATES	678.3 grams	PROTEIN	184.1 grams	FAT	117.6 grams
% CARBOHYDRATES	60.6	% PROTEIN	15.7	% FAT	23.7

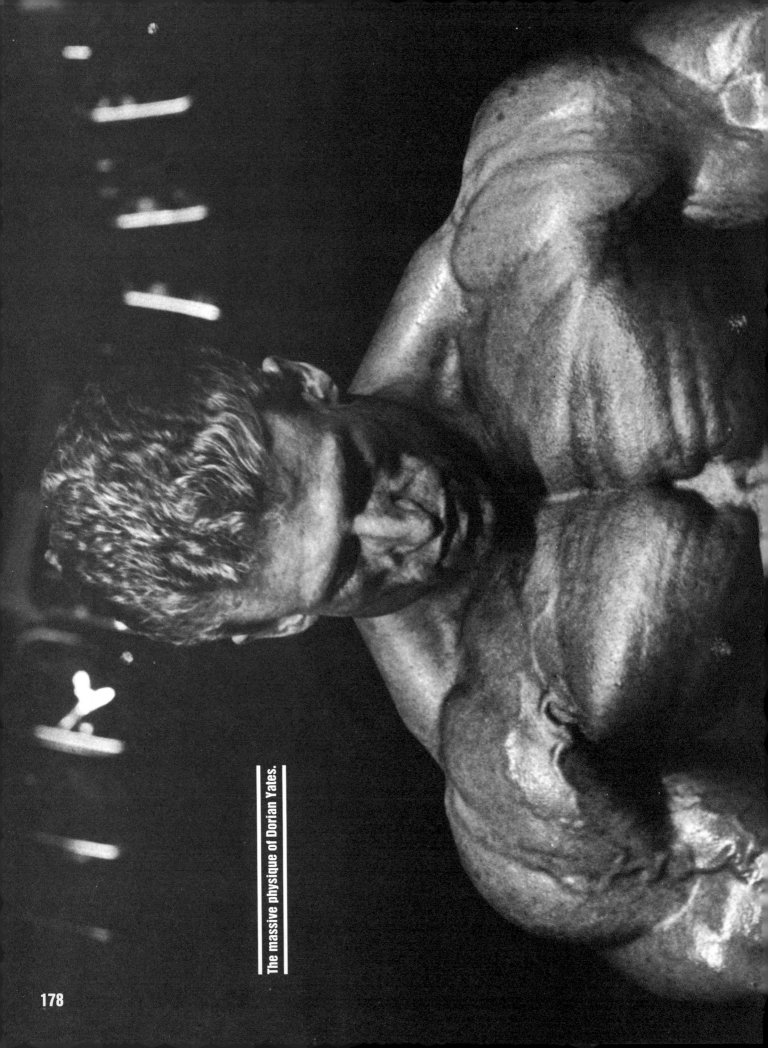

The massive physique of Dorian Yates.

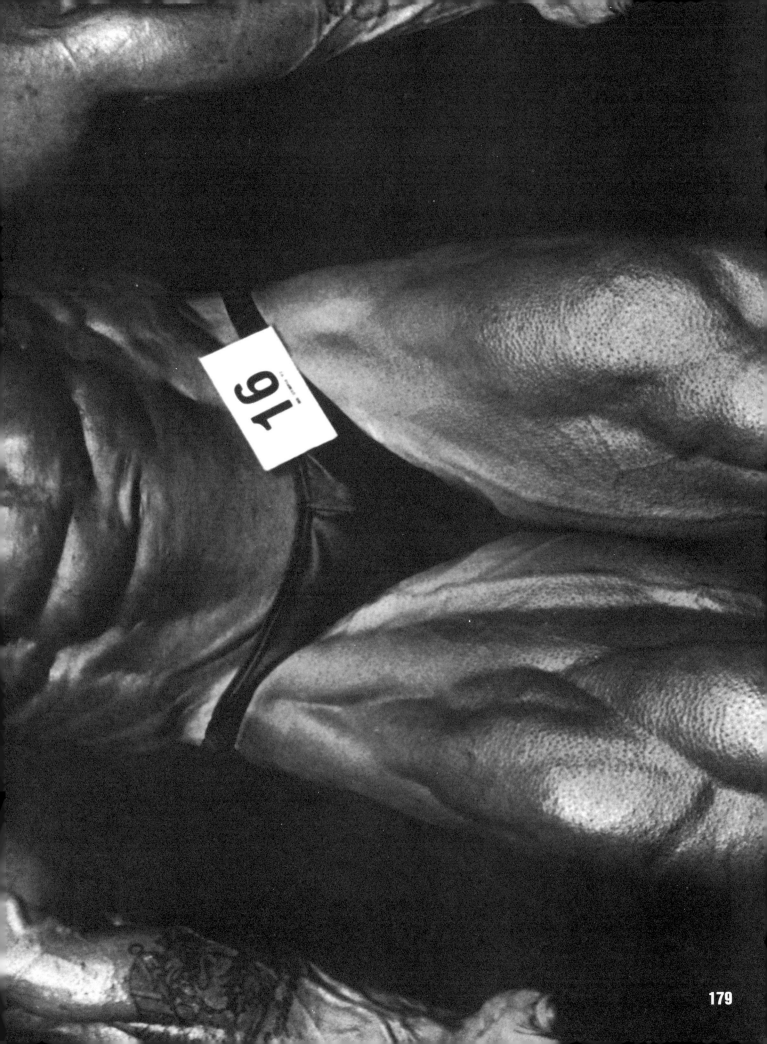

For this last week, I've designed an arm special-ization routine that has never failed to yield signifi-cant results. You'll be shocked by the growth that will occur in your arms. Not only will you be pre-exhausting your biceps and triceps, but you'll be applying a very deliberate style—called 1½-repetitions or 30/30/30—of doing the chin-up and the dip. Get ready to blast your arms to new size. As before, a Monday-Wednesday-Friday schedule is appropriate.

1. 1½-repetition dip. Three exercises make up the triceps and the biceps cycles. You'll need a watch with a second hand to be sure of your slow-ness of movement. Start in the top position of the dip. Lower yourself slowly, inch by inch, in 30 sec-onds. Make a smooth turnaround at the bottom and go back to the top in 30 seconds. Now, do one more negative for 30 seconds. If you can't get each phase exactly in 30 seconds, do the best you can. Move quickly to the triceps extension.

2. Triceps extension with one dumbbell. Pump out as many as possible without cheating. Run back to the parallel bars for the negative dip.

3. Negative dip. Climb up to the top position and lower yourself in 10 seconds. Do as many rep-etitions as you can. Soon you'll become strong enough in this exercise to attach some extra weight around your hips. Take a break and get ready for the biceps cycle.

4. 1½-repetition chin-up. Do the chin-up in a similar manner as the dip: 30 seconds down, 30 seconds up, and 30 seconds down. After you have finished, immediately do the biceps curl.

5. Biceps curl with barbell. You'll have to reduce the weight that you'd normally handle by approximately 30 percent. Try to make the repeti-tions continuous, without pausing at either end. Now hurry back to the chinning bar.

6. Negative chin-up. Get to the top quickly and lower yourself slowly in 10 seconds. Repeat until your lowering time is less than three seconds. Stop and rest for several minutes.

7. Wrist curl with barbell. With an underhand-ed grip on a barbell, be seated and rest your fore-arms on your thighs. Extend and flex your wrists for maximum repetitions.

8. Reverse wrist curl. Use the same position as the wrist curl, except assume an overhanded grip. Also you have to reduce the resistance sig-nificantly.

9. Leg press machine. Go heavy on the leg press, but keep your movement smooth. Do not slam into the lock out. Stop just short of straighten-ing your knees.

10. Leg extension machine. You'll have to re-duce the resistance on the leg extension since you did the leg press before it. Be sure to pause in the top position and do as many repetitions as you can.

11. Leg curl machine. Keep the tension on your hamstrings through the full range of this exercise.

12. Lateral raise with dumbbells. Be sure and lock your elbows on this movement. It makes your deltoids work harder.

13. Bent-kneed sit-up. Curl your shoulders first, then your torso, and touch your chest to your thighs. Lower smoothly and repeat.

GROW: 28-DAY CRASH COURSE
DAYS 22–28: ARM SPECIALIZATION

Exercise	Date Body Weight			
1. 1½-repetition dip				
2. Triceps extension				
3. Negative dip				
4. 1½-repetition chin-up				
5. Biceps curl				
6. Negative chin-up				
7. Wrist curl				
8. Reverse wrist curl				
9. Leg press				
10. Leg extension				
11. Leg curl				
12. Lateral raise				
13. Bent-kneed sit-up				
Name:				

Note: Perform the exercises inside the brackets with no rest in between.

Jeff's muscular size and strength were growing at a rapid rate. Thus, during the last week his calo-ries per day progressed to 4,600. Again, he was consuming daily three large meals and three snacks. One of his final week's menus is as follows:

NAME: Jeff Turner SUNDAY WEEK 4

BREAKFAST	AMOUNT	CALORIES
Eggo waffle, frozen	4	500
Margarine	4 teaspoons	137
Syrup	2 ounces	208
Banana, raw	1 large	117
Skim milk	1 cup	84
Cranberry juice	10 ounces	174

MIDMORNING SNACK		
Raisin bread	2 slices	140
Margarine	2 teaspoons	68
GO! Nutrition Quick-Shake	8 ounces	191

LUNCH		
Garden vegetable soup	2 cups	128
Bread sticks	2	75
Margarine	2 teaspoons	68
Mozzarella cheese, reduced fat	1 ounce	76
Peach, raw	1 medium	42
GO! Nutrition Quick-Shake	8 ounces	191

AFTERNOON SNACK		
Orange sherbet	2 cups	556
GO! Nutrition Quick-Shake	8 ounces	191
GO! Nutrition Quick-Shake	8 ounces	191

DINNER		
Pizza, vegetable topping only	3 slices	797
Tossed salad (raw vegetables only)	1 large	74
Low-calorie salad dressing	2 tablespoons	70
Cranberry juice	8 ounces	139

AFTER-DINNER SNACK		
Cheerios cereal	1 ounce	112
Skim milk	1 cup	84
GO! Nutrition Quick-Shake	8 ounces	191

TOTAL CALORIES = 4,604

CARBOHYDRATES	697.6 grams	**PROTEIN**	183.5 grams	**FAT**	120.9 grams
% CARBOHYDRATES	60.6	**% PROTEIN**	15.8	**% FAT**	23.6

During Week 4 you're going to stimulate your arms to renewed growth.

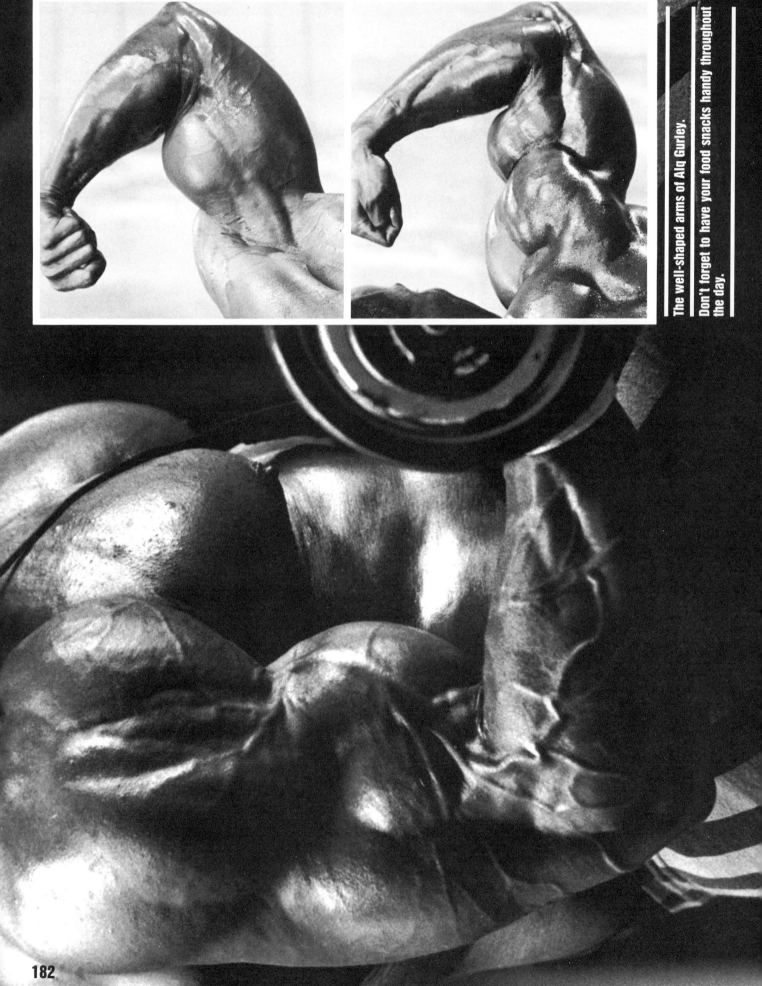

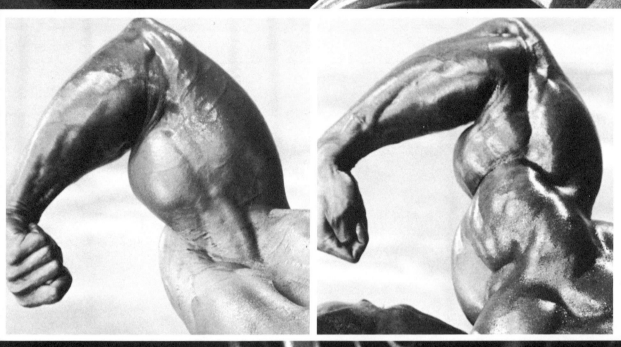

The well-shaped arms of Alq Gurley.

Don't forget to have your food snacks handy throughout the day.

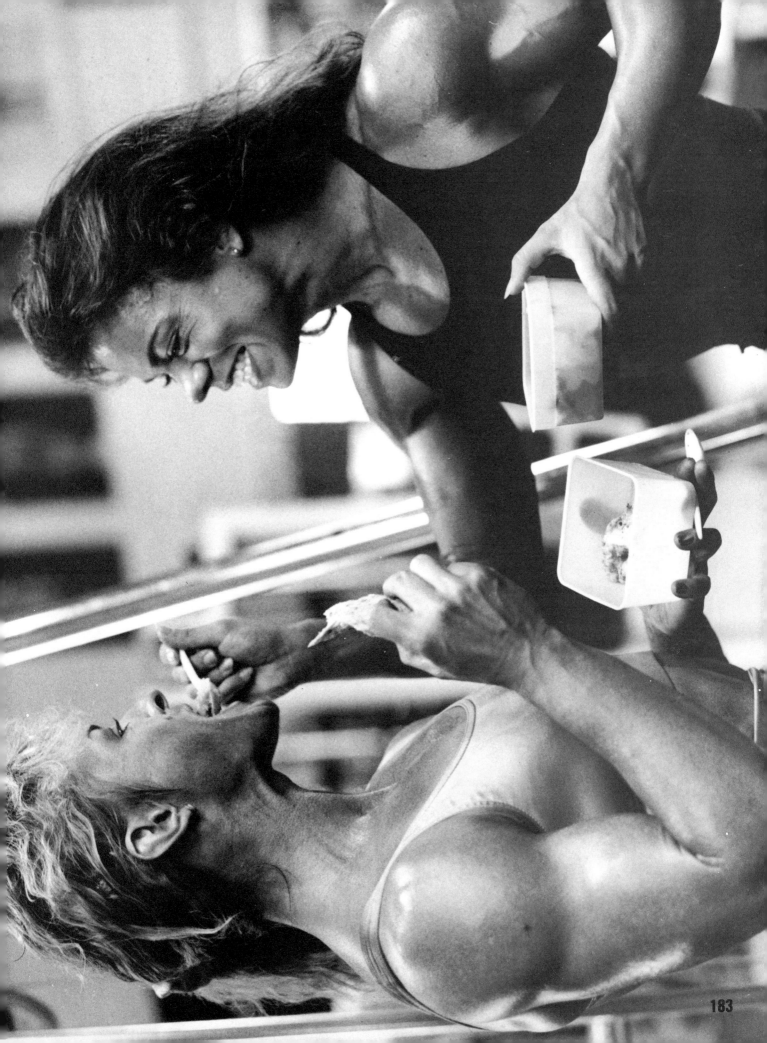

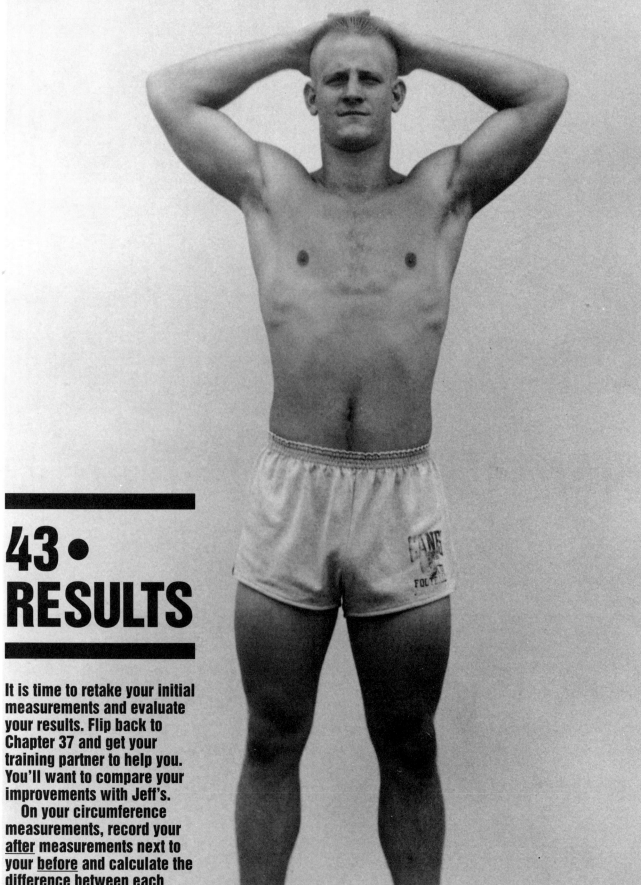

43•
RESULTS

It is time to retake your initial measurements and evaluate your results. Flip back to Chapter 37 and get your training partner to help you. You'll want to compare your improvements with Jeff's.

On your circumference measurements, record your <u>after</u> measurements next to your <u>before</u> and calculate the difference between each pair.

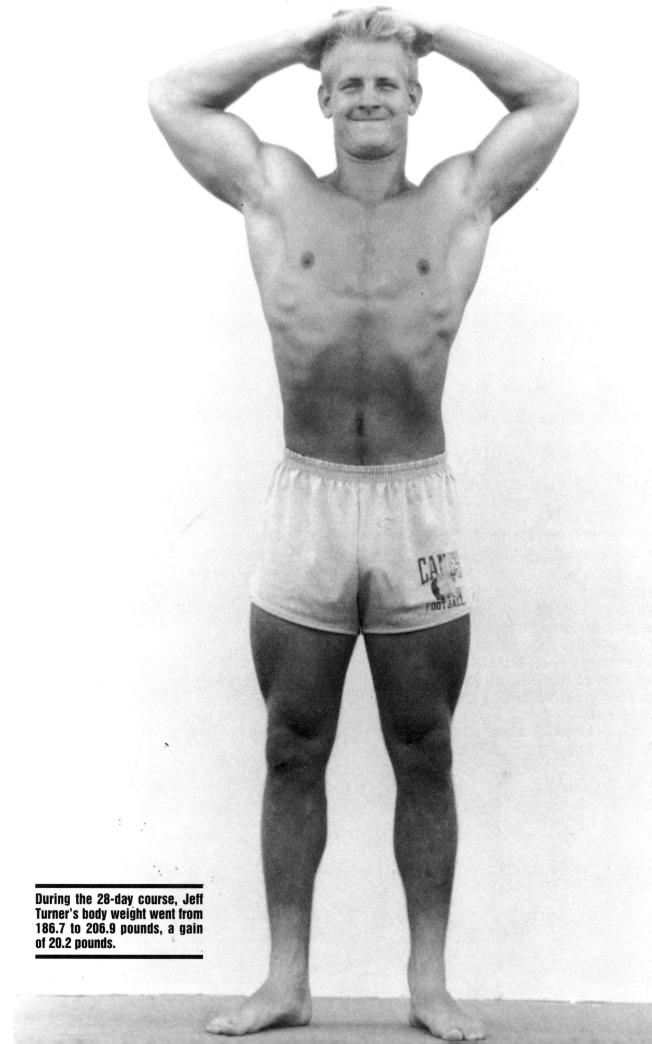

During the 28-day course, Jeff Turner's body weight went from 186.7 to 206.9 pounds, a gain of 20.2 pounds.

JEFF'S MEASUREMENTS			
BODY SITE	BEFORE	AFTER	DIFFERENCE
Neck	15½	15¾	¼
Right upper arm	15⅜	16¼	⅞
Left upper arm	15¼	16⅛	⅞
Right forearm	13	13¼	¼
Left forearm	12½	13	½
Chest	42⅜	44¼	1⅞
Waist	33	33⅞	⅞
Hips	41	41	—
Right thigh	24⅝	26	1⅜
Left thigh	24	25⅝	1⅝
Right calf	15¼	15⅝	⅛
Left calf	15¼	15½	¼
TOTAL INCHES GAINED			8⅞

JEFF'S SKINFOLD VALUES		
	BEFORE*	AFTER*
Chest	3.5	3.5
Waist	15.0	15.5
Thigh	7.0	7.0
TOTAL	25.5	26.0
PERCENTAGE OF BODY FAT	7.0	7.0

* in millimeters

For calculation purposes, the total of Jeff's skinfold values remained basically the same. His percentage did not change—it remained 7 percent. But since his body weight increased significantly, his body fat had to go up slightly, from 13.07 pounds to 14.48 pounds.

In other words, Jeff put on 1.41 pounds of fat. This means that he built 18.79 pounds of muscle. Thus, the 18.79 pounds of muscle plus 1.41 pounds of fat equal 20.2 pounds of body weight.

Jeff and I were both pleased with his overall results, which were noticeable in his before-and-after photographs. Be sure to take another set of pictures of yourself. Your arms, chest, and thighs should be observably bigger!

Note that Jeff's greatest improvements were his upper arms (1¾ inches), chest (1⅞ inches), and thighs (3 inches).

Jeff's body weight and body fat percentage were also interesting. At 19 years of age and a height of 6 feet, Jeff weighed 186.7 pounds at the start of the crash course. At the conclusion of 28 days, he weighed 206.9 pounds. Jeff gained 20.2 pounds, or an average of slightly more than 5 pounds per week.

How much of the 20.2 pounds was muscle? Jeff's skinfold values provided the answer.

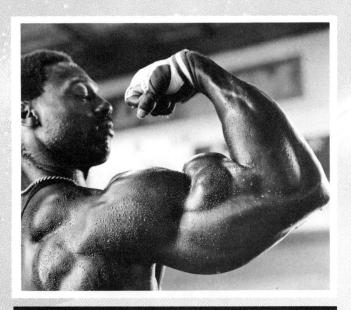

"Magic" is the perfect word to describe Brian Buchanan's right arm.

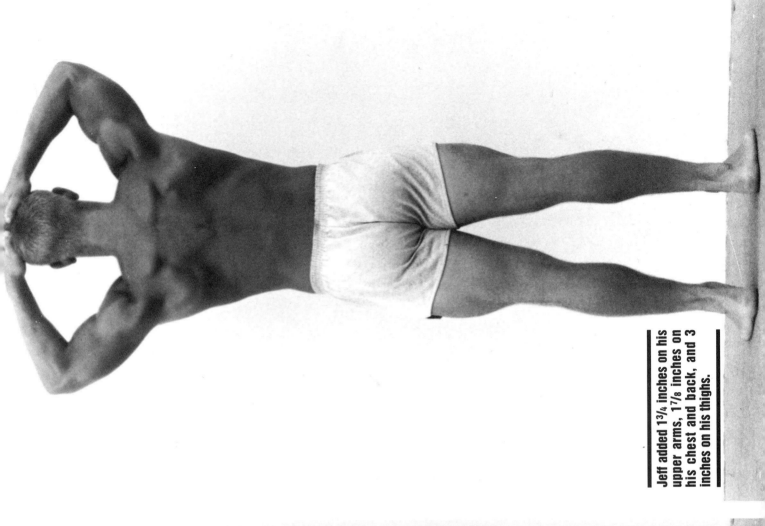

Jeff added 1¾ inches on his upper arms, 1⅞ inches on his chest and back, and 3 inches on his thighs.

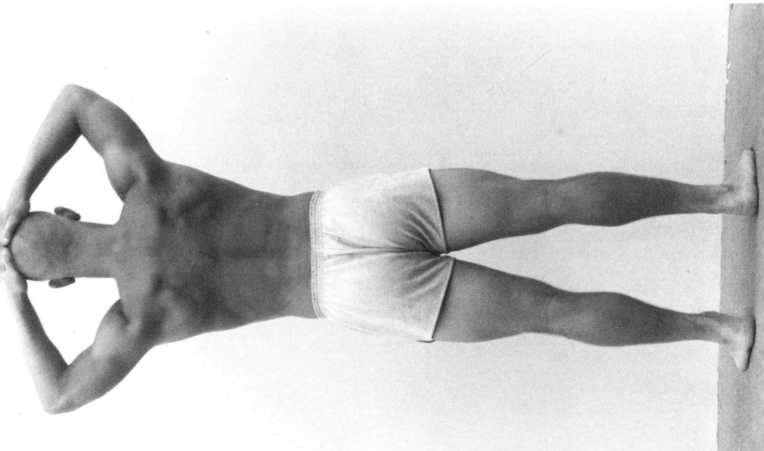

44 • GROW, GROW, GROW!

As a result of the 28-day crash course for getting big, you've gotten a great start on the muscular growth process. But naturally you want more. You want to grow still bigger and stronger, and you want it to happen NOW.

Be patient. The muscular growth process, as you should now realize, takes place in small increments. You grow a little bit each several days. And those little bits can equal a lot in a month or so.

But remember: first you must stimulate growth at the basic cellular level. Only exercise is responsible for this stimulation. Nutrition and rest, while certainly necessary to growth, are not nearly as important as exercise.

To make continual progress in your training, you must understand and apply tried-and-proved guidelines. Here is a brief review of the major ones:

- <u>Hard</u>. Each exercise should be carried to the point of utter failure, where no additional movement is momentarily possible. Most trainees will find it necessary to sit down for a moment after finishing a heavy exercise. If you merely feel like sitting down, then the exercise wasn't hard enough. You should have to sit down to avoid falling down.

- <u>Brief</u> . It is almost impossible for most trainees to work <u>too hard</u>, but it is easily possible for anybody to work <u>too much</u>. In nearly all cases, if the intensity is high enough, one set of any exercise will produce better results than will two or more sets. A workout should not exceed a total of 45 minutes in length. In fact, 30 minutes per workout is an even better goal. The number of exercises per workout should vary from 10 to 20, depending on the equipment available.

- <u>Progressive</u>. Always try to do one more repetition. When you can do 12 or more repetitions correctly, increase the resistance by 5 percent at your next workout.

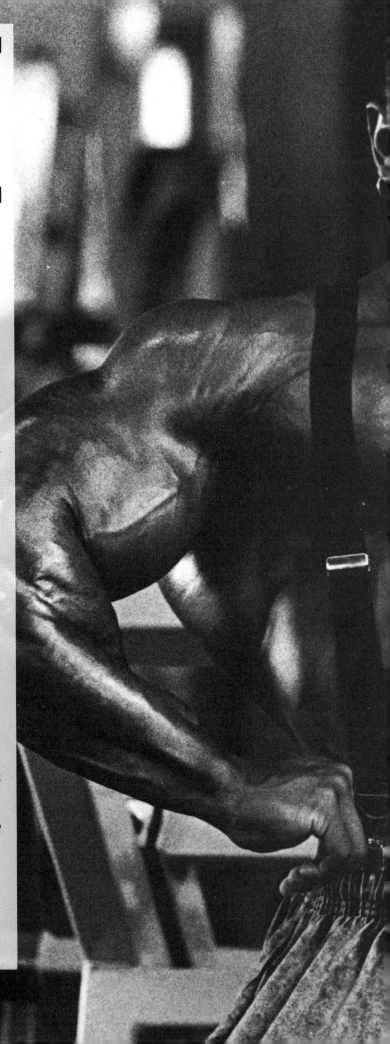

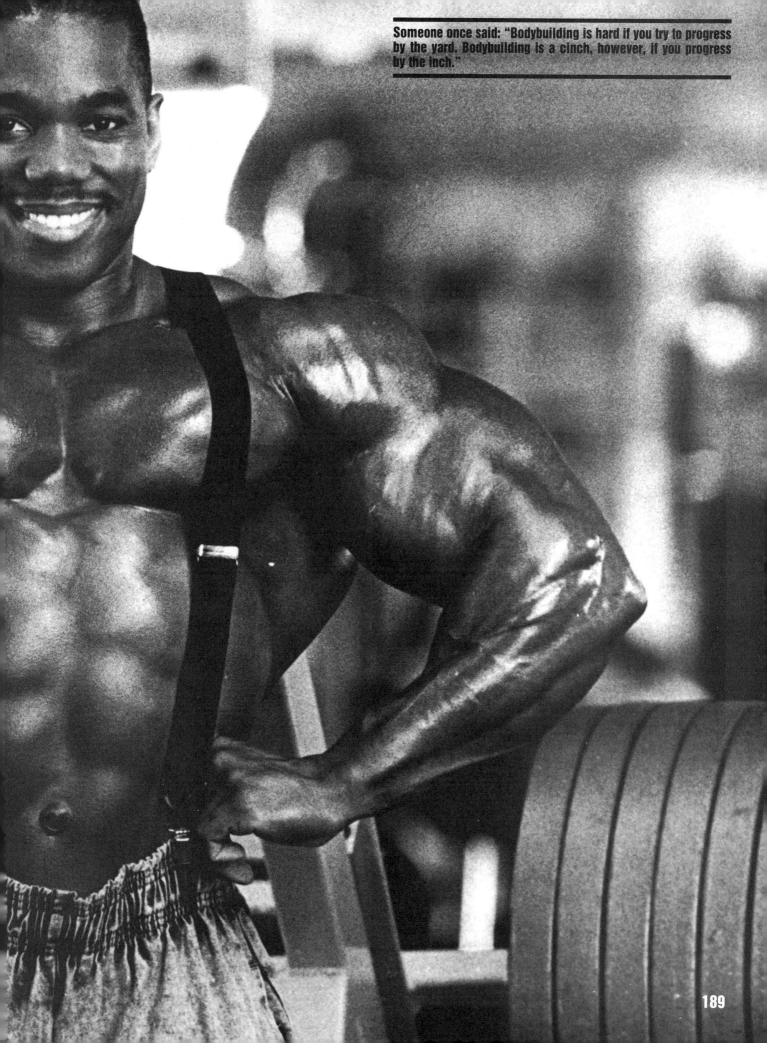

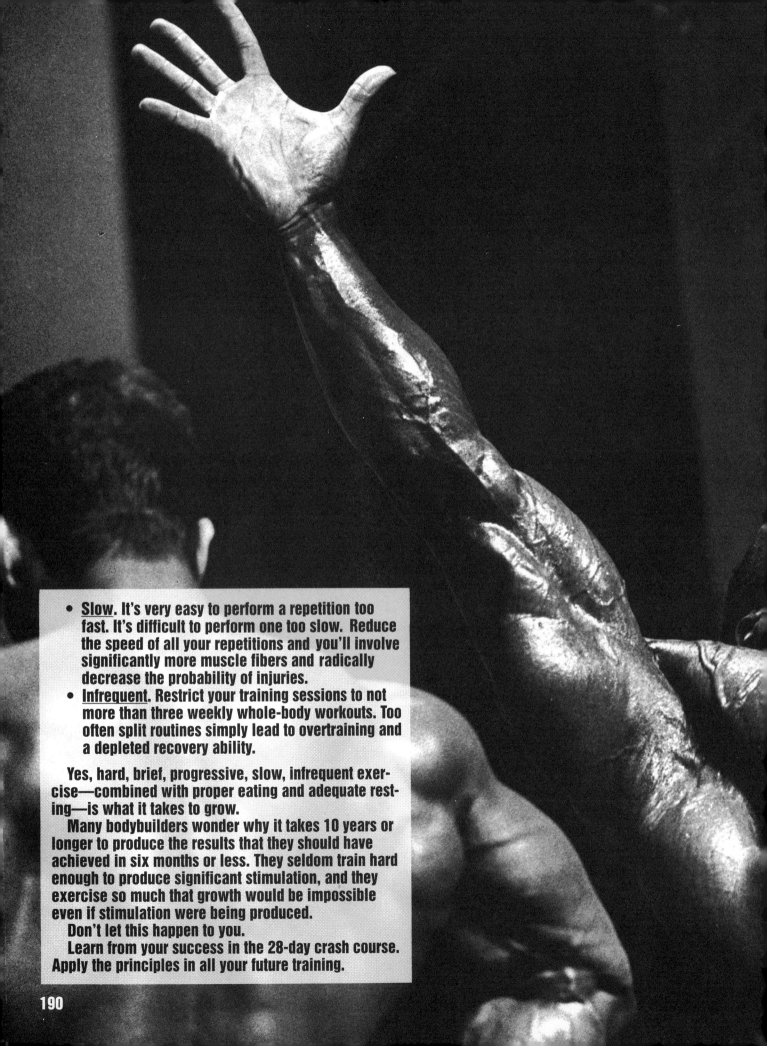

- <u>Slow</u>. It's very easy to perform a repetition too fast. It's difficult to perform one too slow. Reduce the speed of all your repetitions and you'll involve significantly more muscle fibers and radically decrease the probability of injuries.
- <u>Infrequent</u>. Restrict your training sessions to not more than three weekly whole-body workouts. Too often split routines simply lead to overtraining and a depleted recovery ability.

Yes, hard, brief, progressive, slow, infrequent exercise—combined with proper eating and adequate resting—is what it takes to grow.

Many bodybuilders wonder why it takes 10 years or longer to produce the results that they should have achieved in six months or less. They seldom train hard enough to produce significant stimulation, and they exercise so much that growth would be impossible even if stimulation were being produced.

Don't let this happen to you.

Learn from your success in the 28-day crash course. Apply the principles in all your future training.

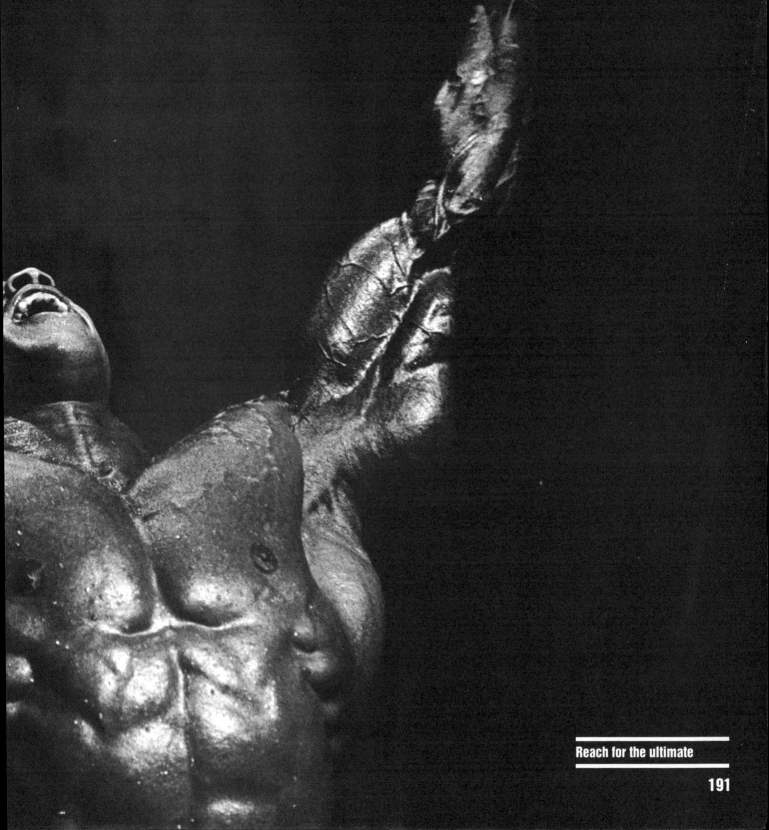

Reach for the ultimate

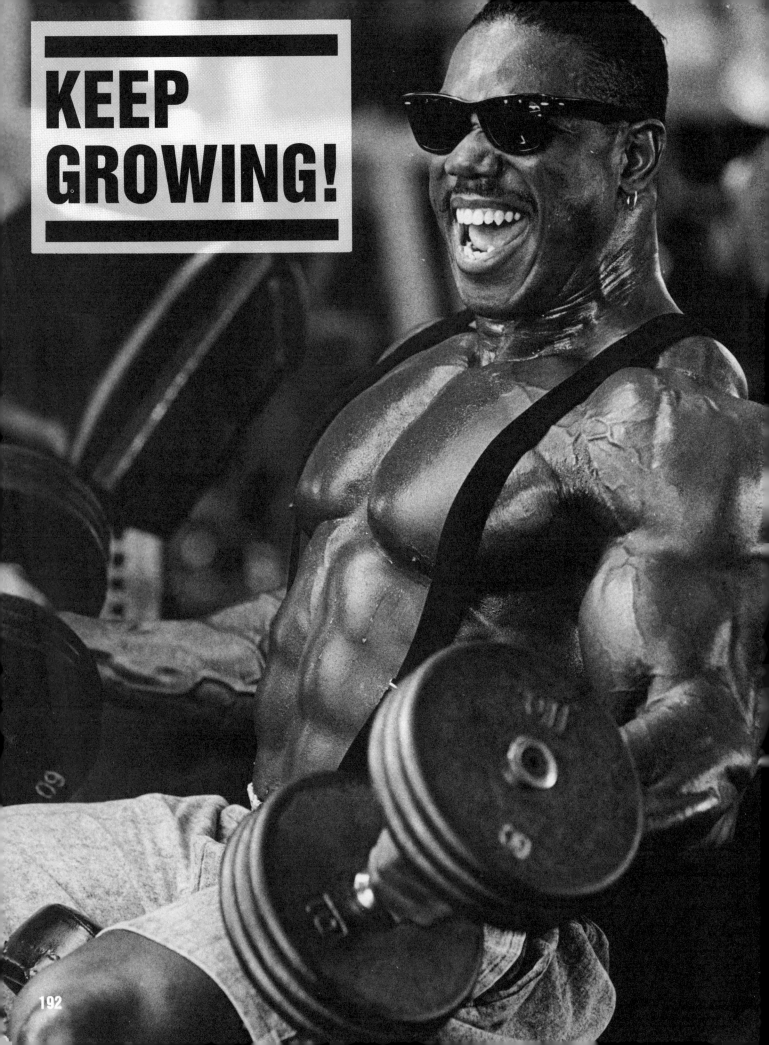

KEEP GROWING!